Introduction

Jim Hotz, M.D. was an inspiration for my novel *Doc Hollywood*, which was made into the major motion picture starring Michael J. Fox. Conspiring to hoodwink Jim into practicing medicine in a south Georgia underserved community was not only fun for me, but has resulted in improved access to health care for tens of thousands of folks. Hopefully my book, *Doc Hollywood*, has motivated other doctors to practice in communities where they are desperately needed.

Jim Hotz and Vic Miller have addressed another important social medical issue in this book. Mixing wit, humor, empathy, and a downright fascinating slice of southern culture, they've created an entertaining tale with a potpourri of colorful characters. On the surface, the story is highly entertaining; however, there is a deeper meaning: American health care is at a fork in the road. Will we select a health care system which is predominantly directed by a free enterprise system? Or will we choose a system which incorporates a priority of providing baseline access to holistic health care for all Americans?

Jim deftly paints a portrait of medicine as we enter the 21st Century. Between the lines he's screaming a warning. He's an advocate for the sensitivity of the medical industry toward the community at large. He obviously understands the contributions of private practitioners, community health centers, and the National Health Service Corps. What he fears is what will happen to these groups as the mega-medical corporations become major players. Is the health care provider of tomorrow going to have any sensitivities to the overall health of the community at large?

This book is a must-read for students and professionals in all areas of medicine. It also provides a unique opportunity for others to get absorbed in a tale rich with intriguing characters living in an unusual culture. I applaud the authors.

-- Neil Shulman, M.D.

Foreword

Neil Shulman first tricked me into coming to Southwest Georgia in 1978. Neil claims this ruse helped inspire his successful novel *Doc Hollywood* that eventually became the hit movie by the same name. Having been victimized once, I should have been wary when fifteen years later Neil drove the two hundred miles from Atlanta to Albany for a "social visit."

"Someone needs to tell the story of rural medicine!" pleaded Neil. "You are the perfect person to tell the rest of the *Doc Hollywood* story!"

One of Neil's great gifts is to inspire others to engage in long-shot crusades, so for people like me Neil's friendship can be a bit of a curse. I had always desired to help develop a rural health care system, and Neil's "encouragement" helped start me toward this goal in the poverty-stricken counties of Southwest Georgia. Neil also knew I harbored a desire to write "the great American novel" and suckered me into a new adventure.

I blame a former instructor, Dr. Pat Carden, for planting the seed for this latest madness. I was an innocent twenty- year-old chemistry geek whom she exposed to the passion of Russian Literature. From Pushkin to Pasternak she stoked the flames. This course was the most influential I took during my four years at Cornell. Chekov became my inspiration. Servant to the rural peasant and artist, he captured Russian humanity to be savored by future readers.

In January of 1993 I started to craft this great work; by March I knew Chekov's position at the top of the heap of physician writers was secure! The great passion that drove my career was the application of the craft of medicine to the rural poor. My novel continually transformed into medical sociology. Neil kept trying to convince me that more health career students would be inspired by a good novel that they "want to read" than any textbook they "have to read." I knew he was right, but in fact I had become after twenty years of seventy-hour weeks a lunchpail-carrying craftsman and not an artist.

Neil and I were both frustrated. I had over thirty-five chapters outlined and a story line that exposed the great themes of rural American medicine today: the need for medical education to produce community responsive family-oriented physicians; the responsibility of health providers to advocate for health delivery systems that care for all in the community, not just the insured; and the unending battle between the for-profit and the not-for-profit providers over whether health care is a "right" or a privilege.

I had the marble out of the quarry, and a rough shape had emerged. Neil convinced me I needed to find a local artist who could sculpt this stone into a thing of beauty. Vic Miller was the name that rushed into my mind. He was perfect for the job--comedian, talented writer, outdoorsman, and brave yet dumb to a fault. Here was a patient of mine who got bitten by a rattlesnake one week after his coronary bypass operation. His cardiac rehab was interrupted by his attempt to capture something interesting for his daughter's "show-and-tell." Who better to take in as a partner in this hopeless crusade?

Three years, a lot of hard work, and quite a bit of fun later our novel is ready. Neil, Vic, and I like to look upon ourselves as the Three Musketeers, but in reality we have performed more like Larry, Curly, and Moe. We are three very different people with very separate lives, but somehow we managed to get this novel out and in a form that makes us very satisfied. We hope the reader will share in our enthusiasm.

The events in this book are based upon my experience in rural medicine. The characters are fictitious. Any resemblance between characters in this book and real individuals is purely coincidental. In particular, any actions by the medical professionals depicted in this novel that vary from social and medical standards are neither endorsed nor condoned by the authors.

This novel is about physicians who serve their rural communities and make a difference. In Southwest Georgia an organization was established to insure there would be sufficient health professionals to meet the medical needs of the community. The Southwest Georgia Area Health Education Center (AHEC) is an outstanding institution, and I would like to recognize the excellent leadership of Pam Reynolds, the executive director, and of Denise Kornegay, the state AHEC program director. Because of the importance of the AHEC organization's work, **the authors of this book are contributing all royalties of this edition to the SOWEGA AHEC in order to establish a program to "grow our own" health professionals for our sector of Georgia.**

    -- James A. Hotz, M.D.

Acknowledgments

I cannot guarantee this novel will entertain you, but hopefully you will find this story as moving and interesting to read as it was to write. I can, however, guarantee that this novel is an accurate account of the complex and revolutionary forces that today are threatening the existence of the "Doc Hollywoods" who, against enormous odds, continue to deliver healing services in poor rural communities. These doctors who share Dr. Stone's values are the true heroes of American medicine

My understanding of rural medicine and the institutions and social currents now impacting it come from my eighteen years experience at Albany Area Primary Health Care, a federally funded Community Health Center, that serves over twenty thousand poor and rural people in Southwest Georgia. I continue to feel a passion about my calling and hope these feelings are transmitted through the pages of this novel. Community Health Centers are powerful institutions that have the potential to transform health care in this country, and I appreciate the opportunity I have been afforded to work at one of the best of these centers. By their design Community Health Centers interact with a wide array of people and institutions both locally and nationally, and from these interactions I have developed the point-of-view presented in this book. Several key concepts of rural medicine are developed, and I would like to acknowledge the origins of these concepts.

For the first time Community Health Centers are featured in American literature. My understanding of these wonderful institutions comes from exposures to the National Association of Community Health Centers, with key contacts being Tom VanCoverden, Dan Hawkins, Dr. Darryl Leong, and Genie Lewis. Community Health Centers are funded through the U. S. Public Health Service, and Dr. Marilyn Gaston, Dr. David Stevens, Dr. David Smith, Dick Bohrer, Marlene Lockwood and Bob Jackson have helped to develope our excellent program through the years.

The National Health Service Corp is also introduced in this novel and has in my opinion been the most successful program yet devised to distribute doctors to areas of need in this country. This program has flourished through the hard work of such people as Dr. Donald Weaver, Dr. Joe Friday, Carolyn Keshinro, and Jesann Hendrix.

The concept of community-oriented rural medical practices was developed through exposure to the National Rural Health Association, especially Jim Bernstein, Tim Size, Bruce Behringer, Donna Williams, and Dr. Tom Dean and through my years of close association with Dr. Doug Skelton and Dr. Alan Dever from the Mercer University School of Medicine, one of the leading producers of rural primary care physicians.

I learned all I know about Public Health from Dr. Paul White, Dr. Paul Newell, Dr. Jim Alley, and Juneile Rhodes. The principles of health planning I used in this book stem from exposure to Alex Kemp, John Perdew, and the innovative staff of the Southwest Georgia Community Health Institute including Paul McGinnis, Dr. Sandy Handwerk, and Dr. Corleen Thompson.

The importance of locally-controlled, not-for-profit hospital boards comes from my experience as Chairman of the Board of Phoebe Putney Memorial Hospital and from exposure to past Chairmen such as Harry Willson, Dr. Chip Moree, Dr. Carl Gordon, and my many other collegues on the board, as well as to contacts with visionary hospital administrators such as Joel Wernick, John Ray, Ed Ollie, Geoffrey Norwood, and Dr. George Chastain.

I received excellent Internal Medicine training under the watchful eyes of Dr. Willis Hurst, Dr. Ken Walker, and of course Dr. Neil Shulman while at Emory University. However, I was not equipped to provide the range of services necessary in rural communities, and in the novel Dr. Stone's "lament of the internist" captures my frustrations. Fortunately one of my greatest career satisfactions was in helping establish the Southwest Georgia Family Practice Residency in Albany. Dr. Lanny Copeland and his staff have created a premier training program. I have had the pleasure to serve on the faculty of this innovative program since its inception, and I believe many of the physician shortages of our part of the state will be remedied by the next generation of "Doc Hollywoods" graduating from this program.

Community Health Centers are presented as one of the solutions to rural medical challenges because of the successes I have witnessed here in Georgia while working at Albany Area Primary Health Care. While the Community Health Center is an excellent vehicle for rural health system development, it is obvious to me that this vehicle is only as good as the people who operate it. My organization has been blessed with a visionary and dedicated staff. Many of the characters in this novel and most of my concepts of health care delivery were inspired by these cherished colleagues. I would like to especially recognize those who have conspired with me over the past decade, often turning down higher paying jobs in more comfortable urban settings: Dr. Bernard Scoggins, Dr. Phil Poulos, Dr. Bill McPeters, Dr. Joyce Neal, Tary Brown, Jim and Bonnie Womack, Pat Hunter, Earlene Burns, and Cindy Leverette. I have learned much from my patients, especially those who have served on our board as chairman including Miriam Worthy, Keith Culpepper, Ida Chambers, Dr. Alfredo Stokes, Otis Hargrove, Annette Bowling, and Larry Willson.

Emergency Medical Services plays a crucial role in any rural health system as Dr. Stone so painfully learns. I developed an early appreciation of the vital role of paramedics from my wife, Trish, who inspired the character Shelley in the novel and who directs the EMS Program at Darton College. Like the other programs in the Allied Health School at Darton, Trish's training is focused on recruiting local talent and pushing them hard so that the resulting health professionals contribute significantly to the local health delivery system. The EMS programs in Baker, Dougherty, and Lee Counties also contributed to the views expressed in the novel.

Besides the medical theme, a major component to Dr. Stone's conversion to rural physician is through his developing appreciation for the beauty and complexity of the southern ecosystem. Considerable inspiration was provided by the Joseph W. Jones Ecological Research Center and its key staff and supporters, including Dr. Lindsay Boring, Bill Walton, Lee Tribble, and Pete McTier.

Ultimately this novel displays that the place "Where Remedies Lie" is in the hearts of local physicians. I could list most of the two hundred physicians on the staff of Phoebe Putney Memorial Hospital for contributing their hearts and souls to the citizens of our region and to the "Hospital with a Heart," but I would like to give special recognition to those who helped in the writing of this novel: Dr. Jeffrey Hoopes, Dr. Chandler Berg, Dr. Carl Gordon, Dr. Chuck Mendenhall, Dr. Phil Roberts, and Dr. Frank Middleton. Tragically, since the writing of this novel one of the finest physicians in our community, Dr. Michael Roberts, met a premature death. He inspired one of the most noble and most colorful characters in this book, which was a way to thank him for all he did for me and my community.

Invaluable assistance in writing and editing this book was provided by Janice Daugherty, William Fuller, Madge Holm, Dr. Henry and Ann Hart, and Julene Roberts. For providing pretty places to work, I am indebted to Mr. and Mrs. "Big" Hart, Sr., and Dr. and Mrs. Tom Johnson. Special thanks to Barb Maidlow who helped to edit this manuscript and to Lou Emond who provided the final layout and edit. A debt of gratitude also to Mike Brooks for the cover design and to Steve Hinton for the cover illustration.

I would also like to recognize the Robert Wood Johnson Foundation's Community Health Leadership Program, especially Catherine Dunham and Susan Bumagin, whose support and recognition helped give me the confidence to proceed with this project.

One theme of this book is a man's search for a "hometown," a wonderful place where personal values are shaped, where self-esteem is instilled by the love of family and friends, and where a child can safely grow and learn to be a responsible, contributing member of society. I have been fortunate in experiencing two great hometowns: my hometown of Fremont, Ohio and my family's hometown of Albany, Georgia. My mother Mary and my wife Trish have provided the love to make the homes, and my good friends in Fremont and Albany provided the caring to make the towns.

Finally I would like to thank our families who tolerated Vic and me during the long hours of this project and who serve as continuing inspirations: our children Stevie, Mary Anne, Jimmy, George, Maisy, Delle, Jimmy M., and Mary Catherine, and our spouses Trish and Claire. Special thanks to Jim and Nancy Bingle who contributed so much to my success in Albany.

-- James A. Hotz, M.D.

Dedicated to the memory of

Dr. Michael H. Roberts

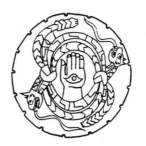

Where Remedies Lie

Our remedies oft in ourselves do lie,
Which we ascribe to heaven.

-- Shakespeare

Chapter One
(Friday 1 April 1983 Grady County, Georgia)

Nurse Holt, black as a plum, settled on her stool at the nurses' station and crackled like a brush fire in her starched whites. "They want you in yonder," she said.

I turned down the hall, pausing at the swinging door of the ER, peaking through the crack, a habit I picked up practicing inner-city medicine in Miami. It's dangerous protocol to charge into an emergency when an argument is going on.

"You stupid son of a bitch," Shelly Farmer told the giant in Stetson hat and khakis, "you still got a choice. You can let Dr. Stone administer antivenin or you can sit there slack jawed while your arm turns black and falls off in your lap."

"Now, now, sweetning. You be a good girl and fetch Carl Hogue. I don't care how drunk he is." Singletree was settled on a chrome stool like a side of beef. He wore a long black pistol, but would have looked dangerous without it. His face was like partially tanned leather stubbled with white whiskers. "I'm right drunk myself for this early in the day, and I ain't in much mood to be fondled by no pissants and dopeheads."

I cringed. I didn't want to enter a room where some redneck had just advised Shelly Farmer, the resplendent paramedic I was in love with, to be a good girl. I didn't mind so much being called a pissant as I minded the syntactical company of Dr. Sherman Flowers, whose history of substance abuse was as well known as my lack of experience.

"Where's your daddy, Buster?" Singletree growled in a voice like corroded plumbing.

Buster Hogue, the athletic ambulance driver who also carried a torch for Shelly, didn't seem put off by the patient's aspersions toward his father. He had retreated, with Frog Hullet, over by the autoclave and out of the path of Shelly's anger. I recognized Frog as the town gopher.

"One these days somebody gone come out that door and bust you flat," snapped Nurse Holt from behind me. I jumped, bumping the door. Over the ruckus I hadn't heard her rustle up or seen her reflected in the chrome push plate. "Who's the giant?" I whispered.

"Hackamore Singletree. He the principal of the junior high," she said.

"He's what? . . . Are you sure?"

Her eyes widened and her pink lower lip emerged. "What you think, I'm line?"

"What's wrong with him?"

"He been snakebit again."

1

"He doesn't look much like a principal."

"How do a principal look?"

Buster rolled an IV tree beside Singletree, unbuttoning a shirtsleeve and skinning it back over a thick simian forearm covered with coarse black hair. "Dr. Hogue's unavailable," Buster was saying, grinning impishly. I liked Buster, although he was a rival of sorts. He'd be fine if his father would stop pushing him so hard.

Nurse Holt opened the door, and I followed her in. "You need to know," she said, "you're his third choice for a physician. He went to the vet first, but Dr. Hartwell wouldn't treat him. You also need to know he has never paid a medical bill in his life.

"Now THERE's an ungrateful practitioner who ought to be censured by his tribe," Singletree drawled. "I swapped him out as fine a liverspot pup as there was in Dixie, which he ruint by making him gun-shy. Now he's got too highborn to administer to the infirm." Singletree's speech was spiked with unusual vocabulary, giving it a strangely archaic and erudite character, but rough hewn as though he'd taught himself from antique books by firelight. I later learned he was one of those unique insomniacs addicted to print, that he read indiscriminately everything he got his hands on.

"Said he ain't supposed to treat humans," Frog said.

"Hackamore's not human," Shelly snapped. "Take him back over there and tell Hartwell I'll pay cash money to have his ass put to sleep."

"The truth of it is he ain't supposed to charge for treating humans," Singletree said.

When he turned to face me, I noticed his misshapen face. The lower half of one side of his head was twice the size of the other. "You're Stone," he said.

"The resident pissant," I added coldly.

I put on my latex gloves and gently touched is swollen jaw with my forefinger. "Does that hurt?"

"No," he grinned.

"That's his chaw, Otis," Shelly said.

"What?"

"You're probing his chewing tobacco."

A sound like a punctured truck tire escaped Nurse Holt. She left the ER, returning to her nurses' station.

"Where did the snake bite you?"

"Toa Swamp."

"Where on your body?"

Hack held up a thumb, the end of which was swollen the size of a golf ball. I examined the discolored digit and found red streaks running up his wrist and forearm. "Take off your shirt," I told him. The big man winced as he moved his arm. "Were you bitten anywhere else?"

"My ankle, she hit me there and latched on. She caught my thumb when I pulled her off. Tried to hang on there too. I got to jumping around like a man trying to throw off a piece of flypaper."

I squatted to examine his ankle. The linoleum smelled of Lysol, which Nurse Holt preferred over more modern disinfectants. I removed his brogan and slit the leg of his trousers with my scissors. His ankle was swollen like a bota bag, yellow and purple, with two puncture wounds about a centimeter apart where the swelling was greatest. There was only one fang mark on his thumb.

"Well, it look like a snakebite to you, Doc?"

"That or a vampire."

I locked my hands behind my lab coat and cleared my throat, getting professional. "Did you bring in the snake that bit you?" I asked, nodding at the brown paper bag in Frog's lap. "Let's see." Standard medical procedure was to identify the reptile as poisonous, since large doses of antivenin were themselves dangerous. Although I wasn't sure I could identify a snake that didn't have rattles on the tip of its tail, I remembered from med school that poisonous snakes have triangular heads. Frog opened the bag, revealing a half-quart Mason jar of clear liquid. "That ain't the snake," laughed Hack. "That's *my* antidote. The snake's out in the pick-up. Get the snake, Frog."

He grinned, "I didn't mean nothing personal with the *pissant* stuff. Except Henry Hartwell treats about 500 snakebit dogs to ever one human Doc Hogue gets. I'll venture that this one is about your first bona fide case."

"That's true, but I was in the Boy Scouts, and I'm certified to treat human beings, not dogs. That's a distinct advantage over the vet."

"Well, dogs and men are close enough. In the long haul, a few minor anatomical dissimilarities set aside, the main difference between your *canis familiaris* and your *homo sapiens* is a dog's got a better sense of direction. A dog ain't as likely to spend as much time lost, which broaches the question, what the hell are you doing in Grady, Georgia, now that you graduated the Boy Scouts?"

"Mechanical malfunction and love. My car broke down on the interstate, and I became enamored of that resplendent paramedic over there. I'm basically a victim of circumstance." This was heavy truth spoken lightly, and the whole town knew it.

"She *is* a pretty thing, ain't she?" Hack said. Shelly squinted balefully at us both.

Suddenly, outside the ER we heard commotion. "You get out of here with that snake RAT now!" Nurse Holt screamed from the front desk.

"The doc told me to brang him in," Frog protested. Holt followed him into the

ER He carried a writhing four-and-a-half foot snake the circumference of a soup can. "Doctor!" she cried, "Doctor Stone!"

The headless neck dripped bright drops of blood that splattered the linoleum. The thick body contracted and surged, lashing violently. The tail blurred gray, filling the ER with a dry buzz that made the hair rise on my arms and the back of my neck. I sprung to my feet.

"It's still alive!" I screamed.

"Naw, she's dead," laughed Hack. "Her head just ain't been able to tell her ass end yet, it being on the other side of town. Look at her still trying to pop poor old Frog."

Frog stood before us deadpan and miserable. He had splotches of wet red on his cheek and his T-shirt where the headless snake had struck him. His wide mouth and protuberant eyes recalled a story in which a fairy princess kisses a frog, transforming it into a prince with amphibian features.

"Go ahead and look her over, Doc." Hack urged. "I believe you'll find this snake here is a fine specimen of *Crotalus adamanteus*--in her ninth molt, woefully interrupted by yours truly. Don't worry about all that fuss. She's got a highly organized reflex nervous system, most of which ain't in her head."

"Uh, you can take the snake out of the ER now, Frog."

"Wait a minute, Doc," said Hack. "Take a close look. That's as good a color as you'll see on a diamondback. Look how bright the dorsal markings are."

If I could have put aside my deeply rooted, perhaps innate, fear of reptiles, I'd have appreciated the snake as a beautiful creature. But I couldn't put prejudice aside. This snake was as loathsome to me as the one that tempted Eve, but I was also curious. Shed skin hung like cellophane from the front half of its body. "What's that peeling off?"

"That's her slough." Hack said. He removed some of the opalescent skin and pointed out clear cuticles, like contact lenses, where the reptile had shed the cloudy membrane covering its eyes. The new skin was marked with black and yellow diamonds. Hack held a coil out for me to touch, and I reached out reluctantly, expecting the snake to be slimy, but the plates and beaded scales were cool and dry like brightly polished jewelry.

"They can't see good when they're molting, and it makes them testy. Of course, this one could see fine."

So this redneck was also an articulate authority on poisonous reptiles. He seemed oblivious to the fact that even now a deadly hemotoxin was spreading toward the lymph nodes of his armpit and groin. I started an IV and sent Mrs. Holt to the refrigerator for snake serum.

"Well," Hack said with a touch of alcoholic remorse, "I ought to be ashamed for killing a pretty thing like that."

4

"How can you tell it's a female?"

"The females are wider at the hips." He winked at Shelly, who glared back. "And they wiggle when they crawl."

"Hackamore is very proficient at hunting down beautiful creatures, like deer, and eating them," Shelly said.

"Why'd you want to eat something ugly, sweetening?" asked Hack. "How long can you keep pretty eating turnip bottoms and turkey necks? You are what you eat, Miss Shelly. Now, what you been eating that makes you so hostile to your old buddy Hack?" Although he bantered with Shelly, I knew snakebite was extremely painful. His rictal grin was like a chamois twisted on a stick. I gave him a shot of morphine.

"How's the pain?"

He leaned toward me. "It hurt so bad," he whispered, "I wanted to slam my dick in the door to divert my attention, but moonshine's a good general anesthetic, don't you think?"

"The worst."

I started another vial of antivenin. I couldn't guarantee that Singletree wouldn't get serum sickness, an allergic reaction to the antivenin, no matter how carefully I regulated the dosage. I was worried about the red streaks up the inside of his arm, and his lower leg looked like Alley Oop's. I was prepared to administer massive doses of the serum. I wasn't worried that we'd run out; hospitals in the deep South carry lots of antivenin. I gave Hack nine vials in all.

"Hey Doc, you better slack off on that joy juice," he finally said. "That snake weren't but half grown, and you've give me enough to cure a hit from a king cobra."

"Young snakes are more potent," I ventured with unsure authority. Frog nodded in agreement.

"Well, I heard *that*! I used to be more potent myself." He eyed Shelly, who stormed out of the ER whooshing through the doors. "She's right pretty when she's mad, ain't she, Doc."

"Yes, and she's a lot prettier when she's mad at somebody besides me. How'd you know this is the snake's ninth molt?" I asked.

"She's got eight rattles. They add a rattle ever time they shed."

"The dust off them rattles will blind you," Frog added.

"Aw Frog," said Hack. "Don't be feeding the doc none of that bullshit."

"It will too," Frog pouted.

"What took you into the Toa Swamp in the first place, Mr. Singletree?"

"*Mr.* Singletree's my daddy," he grinned, flashing long teeth. "My name's Hack. I was down there tracking the Gatorman."

"The *Gatorman*? You wouldn't pull a Yankee pissant's leg, would you,

Hack." The Gatorman was a swamp monster, a creation that frightened children and enriched the fantasies of the local imagination. It left monstrous footprints, wheezing and stinking as it walked, a sort of south Georgia Big Foot or Sasquatch. Like with any other hoax, rumors of sightings were epidemic, yet still no sober and responsible adult had testified to an actual first hand sighting.

"Upon my honor," he smiled, "something strange is in yonder."

"Have you found anything?"

"Some foot tracks I couldn't figure out."

"Did you photograph them or make a plaster of Paris mold?"

"What for?"

"So others would believe you."

"Why should I give a whispering shit what other people believe?"

Chapter Two

Well, what have you got against Hackamore Singletree," I asked Shelly as she undressed for bed. I'd tried to admit him to the hospital but he refused, insisting that he had to be home before dark.

Shelly Farmer was the first attractive girl I'd met since my Porsche broke down on I-75 and had to be dragged to this backwoods municipality by Melvin Dryden's Garage and Wrecker Service. Discovering I was an M.D., Melvin refused to honor my credit cards until he cleared me through Commissioner Worthy, and I got stuck between an internal medicine residency in Miami and an Atlanta interview for an oncology fellowship. I was detained by a combination of uncanny events, which I later discovered to be elements of a canny and well orchestrated plot to shanghai a doctor, any doctor, into a disastrously underserved county. I missed my interview and became stuck in time in Grady, Georgia (pronounced Jawja) with no other prospects but working at the local hospital to pay room, board and automotive expenses. I further complicated my predicament by falling rather helplessly in love with the ambulance driver--oops, *paramedic*-- but there were moments when my lack of direction didn't seem all bad.

"Well, what?" I asked her again.

"Against Hack Singletree?" she asked. "You mean besides his being a disgusting, dangerous, drunken redneck lout?" Shelly reached behind her back to unhook her bra, a gesture that made me suddenly short of breath. I'd once playfully asked her why she hadn't joined her feminist sisters in discarding the *symbolic yoke of male oppression.* "Because this yoke is what's holding my tits up," she answered. "Get real, Stone." Shelly wasn't an excessively symbolic person. I wasn't tempted to dismiss her aversion to Singletree because he represented some vague notion of displaced male values. Shelly's dislike for things was grounded in facts not abstractions.

"Dangerous?" I challenged. "I admit he gives off a foreboding initial impression, but he seems sort of, uh, benign, a gentle giant."

"You just haven't had to patch up somebody he's pistol-whipped yet."

"Pistol-whipped? You're kidding. "

"I'm *not* kidding."

"Who did he pistol-whip?"

"*Whom.*"

"*Whom* did he pistol-whip?

"Wilkin Wright for openers and Marvin, Wilkin's brother."

"Why?"

"The stories vary, but he was drunk when he did it. Even Rooster Bootman, the sheriff, admits that. Of course, it's hard to catch Hack doing anything when he's not drunk, unless it's sleeping. Being drunk still serves as a justifiable excuse for sociopathic behavior in Grady.

"What do you mean *even* Rooster Bootman?"

Shelly started on her nails. She was naked, with the covers pulled up to her waist. She began filing her nails, which wobbled her breasts, nearly mesmerizing me away from the subject of Hackamore Singletree.

"Hack and Bootman are old pals. When Wilkin's daddy, Karl Wright, demanded Hack be arrested for assault and battery, Bootman took Hack home with him. They drank moonshine and played poker until things settled down. Bootman is supposed to have said in Hack's defense, 'He ain't assaulted nobody didn't need it.' The Wrights dropped the charges after Hack sent word he was going to kill all Karl Wright's children except Beulah. There aren't but the three. He meant he was going to kill Wilkin and Marvin. That's just the way he talks. He said there wasn't anything wrong with Karl Wright's two boys that killing wouldn't cure and he had some patented medicine."

"Is Beulah Dr. Lee Bob Parker's wife?"

"The same."

I knew about Dr. Lee Bob. When Dr. Hogue fired Parker from the Trafford staff for assaulting a female patient, Karl Wright made his son-in-law director of the Wright's health-care-for-profit nursing home, Lilies of the Field--which looked like a place Dante assigned the lost and the damned.

"What inclined Singletree to spare Beulah?" I asked.

"It's against Hack's morals to kill a woman except in self defense. Besides, Beulah and Hack were, uh, consorts once, probably still are behind Lee Bob's back. Or with his grudging consent."

"You Southerners are a chivalrous lot."

"Hack and Beulah have been at it a long time. They've carried on for decades, whenever Beulah comes into heat."

"Why doesn't Lee Bob do something about it?"

"What could he do? Hack and Beulah are hard subjects to do anything about individually. Together...well, want a scenario? Get this: Dr. Lee Bob Parker barges into the Magnolia Motel and surprises his wife in the hairy arms of Hack Singletree in full and mindless rut. Hack and Beulah, who haven't even bothered to lock the door, finish the orgasmic throes of primordial lust and turn to the astonished Lee Bob. Beulah etches the picture glass window with maniacal laughter while Hack, squinting through puffy eyes, puts on his boots to 'stomp a trench in Lee Bob's cloven ass.'"

"Did this really happen? Or is it your allegorical way of saying Beulah and Hack don't take Dr. Parker seriously," I smiled.

She hoisted her eyebrows. "Does anyone take him seriously?"

"He's a serious danger to patients."

"Well, you'll meet Beulah at her daddy's shindig, where we'll introduce you to all the health care hotshots in southwest Georgia." Beulah Parker was on the Trafford Memorial hospital board, where (according to Shelly) she has fornicated herself into power over all the members except Miss Ida. Miss Ida was the leonine, 70-year-old, no-nonsense wife of Commissioner Worthy. She drank her whisky neat, cussed like a stevedore, and harbored a relentless civic-minded resolution to keep me in Grady County against my will. Because of Ida Worthy, the whole town kept a running tab on everything I needed to be comfortable and stranded here. Nobody would accept my credit cards unless she approved each purchase, and the bank wouldn't approve a loan for anything that hinted of transiency. Three things kept me in Grady. I was broke, lovesick, and professionally aimless now that my oncology residency at Emory had been filled by someone else.

"Are there children?" I quipped of the Parker-Singletree triangle. I pictured a horse-toothed, outsized spawn of Hack booting Lee Bob out of his own baronial home. "Is the Parker household blessed with offspring?"

"It's rumored that Beulah's seminal fluids are spermicidal."

Shelly began painting her fingernails with polish bright as partridge berries.

"Somehow, I just can't picture your friend Singletree hurting anybody. Course, I can't picture him in love either."

"He's capable of both," Shelly said, shuddering, "but I'm not sure I'd call the knotting and gendering those two practice love. But Hack's gotten to be bad medicine. His alcoholism has progressed and his politics have polarized. He's not somebody you want to cross."

She paused, becoming more serious. "Dr. Hogue had to sew Wilkin's nose back on," she said. "If you'd seen Wilkin's nose, you wouldn't have any trouble picturing your Hack Singletree hurting somebody."

"This is medieval. Did Singletree bite Wilkin's nose off or chop it off with an ax?"

"The front sight of his pistol tore it off when Hack backhanded him."

"Why did he backhand him?"

"Wilkin interrupted Hack, who was trying to collect evidence Marvin swallowed. Hack claims he was trying to make Marvin vomit up a rock of crack cocaine. Hack had to yank his pistol out of Marvin's mouth to hit Wilkin." Shelly splayed her fingers at arm's length, cocking her head. Now this was Southern Gothic. I was lying in bed naked with a beautiful paramedic who told horror stories while doing her nails.

"He was gagging him with a pistol?"

"He wouldn't use his finger because he was afraid Marvin would bite him.

9

Hack thinks Marvin has gay pneumonia, AIDS."

"Does he?"

"How should I know? Hack thinks all dopeheads have AIDS. The region's had two cases this year. Seven have been reported in Georgia by the Center for Disease Control in Atlanta. Paul Dudley--he's the regional health director--says that crack cocaine will bring an AIDS epidemic."

This was 1983. AIDS was a brand new pestilence. The first case was diagnosed in San Francisco in '81, a year of ominous attempted assassinations of presidents and popes and the successful murder of 28 black children in Atlanta.

"But isn't crack smoked? AIDS is transferred by contaminated syringes."

"And sex. Dudley's got Hack convinced that crack houses are hotbeds of sexual promiscuity and social disease, especially syphilis. Group sex is common in crack houses where prostitutes, dopeheads, and chicken heads swap sex for drugs."

"So crack's hit Dixie, too."

"It's catching on like MTV and the Sony Walkman. Hack claims he was trying to make a citizen's arrest and stop drug traffic at the junior high. He knocked out three or four of Marvin's teeth, jabbing around, trying to plumber up that rock of cocaine. Hack told the judge he was exercising a contractual option of an agreement he had made with Wilkin and Marvin Wright, whom he had allegedly warned: 'I find any more drugs over at the junior high school, and it no more than a roach of rabbit tobacco, I'm gone rip off your heads and piss down your throats.' Or words to that effect." She fanned her nails, then rested her chin on her knees and started on her toes.

"This is the principal of the junior high?" I could smell the acetone in Shelly's nail polish remover. It was more or less the fruity smell on the breath of diabetic patients in diabetic ketoacidosis.

"Such as he is. He doesn't talk quite so rough around women and children. I hear all the Hackamore Singletree stories from the ambulance drivers and orderlies, where I transcend the barriers of gender." She batted her eyelids and smiled. "Hack's mamma raised him right, or tried to, and to give a devil his due, Grady Junior High students somehow do well on national exams. Don't ask me how." Shelly spread her toes to paint them.

"He can't be as bad as you fashion him then," I said. I admired the way Shelly could splay her toes. Men can't do it without their great toe turning upward and their other toes curling under. Early in life women must develop the vestigial muscles required to fan their toes, that or it's an anatomical distinction.

"He's pretty bad. What infuriates me most is his utter lack of ambition. He has a high mental aptitude, and he's the best read redneck in Georgia. But he is exactly that. A redneck. His idea of culture is sitting around a fire between midnight and dawn with his redneck buddies, drinking illegal whiskey, swapping lies and listening to a howling pack of bluetick and redbone hounds swarm the Swamp of Toa."

"How idyllic. Sounds like you've been there."

She held her ankles, leaned forward, pursed her lips and blew. "I've been there plenty of times."

"With Hack?"

"With Hack. And others, but Hack's drinking has increased his paranoia and his loutish behavior. He's always been a hick. He's not interested in venturing outside the county line. Of course, he had to go in the Army when everybody in Grady got drafted, but he came home after two years and hasn't left home since."

"He went off to college, didn't he? He's a principal."

"The fool bought his credentials from a diploma mill in Alabama after he got conscripted to principal. Nobody else would take the job. He never attended college, but he's a reader. Not to better himself. He can't help it, it's a disease. The bastard is addicted to print. He'll read a catsup bottle, an Elizabethan sonnet, or the yellow pages, whatever's there." She paused, watching me. "What in the *hell* are you doing?" she demanded.

"What do you mean?"

"You're staring at your foot and straining your mouth."

"Nothing. I was just thinking that this is some kind of pillow talk," I said, rubbing a cramp from my little toe. I kissed her shoulder, which was strong and brown, a swimmer's shoulder. Shelly stayed in shape by swimming upstream in the Kinchafoonee Creek, an appropriate exercise for someone with Shelly's disdain for traditional female roles.

"You brought it up. Hack Singletree is the last subject I want in my prenuptial bed." She tilted her head to offer her neck, keeping her tacky fingers and toes safely out of the way.

"What subject?" I mumbled, nuzzling her clavicle.

Chapter Three

My unsolicited mentor Dr. Carl Hogue, the crusty family practitioner who'd provided the mainstay of Grady County medicine for the past forty years, insisted that Shelly and I attend Karl Wright's cocktail party, which was to feature some of the foremost shakers and movers in the medical community. We took the ambulance and met Dr. and Mrs. Hogue and their son Buster, an ambulance driver and ER orderly with vague, paternally imposed ambitions of someday becoming a neurosurgeon. He was shaped more or less like an upright freezer with long blond hair, and he was enamored of Shelly, therefore cool to me, but I liked him anyway.

I hadn't even packed a suit for my trip to Atlanta. I'd expected to scout out the styles on Peachtree and buy appropriately before my interview. Although still naive about the deep South, I was savvy enough to know that although Miami and Atlanta are less than 800 miles apart, they are as different as Boston from Tangier.

We passed beneath the columns of Wright's antebellum mansion, finding ourselves surrounded by black tuxedos, taffeta, and crystal. I felt comically out of place in the white dinner jacket that had belonged to Shelly's cremated father. I'd had to belt in the roomy trousers with the cummerbund so that they bunched in the back and the satin trouser stripe migrated backwards from the sides of the legs. The only other white coats belonged to the waiters and bartenders. Still, I was less conspicuous than the group I walked in with. Dr. Hogue sported a double breasted suit he'd carried off to med school, and Mrs. Hogue wore an actual magnolia blossom in her hair.

What we lacked in style, we made up for in accessibility to Nurse Holt, who was minding the shop alone. Buster, in a plaid coat and white bucks, carried a two-way radio, and Shelly had her beeper clipped into the cleavage of her evening dress. At least I blended in with the servants.

I had strict instructions from Mrs. Hogue to keep Dr. Hogue from getting drunk. I had originated the order myself, reducing his alcohol to one ounce per day after he'd suffered a heart attack on January 31. I now confronted the stark and ironic reality of trying to enforce a doctor's order on a doctor. Hogue charged the bar like the proverbial mule homing in on the barn. Before I could catch him, a Flint radiologist handed me his glass and asked me to refresh his martini. "Go easy on the gin, son. I'm on call," he said.

"That's a good way to mingle," whispered Shelly. "You're not going to do it, are you?"

"What?"

"Fetch that jerk's drink."

"Why not?"

"You'll sacrifice your station?" she smiled.

"What station?"

The bar was set up on the terrace, in the soft light of Japanese lanterns. I ordered the doc's martini, an orange juice and champagne concoction called a mimosa for Shelley, and a beer for myself. Ignoring the black bartender, two humorless thugs in designer jeans (I deduced them to be Wilkin and Marvin Wright) elbowed their way to the backside of the bar, removed a quart of tequila and disappeared across the lawn. Waiting for the drinks and listening to the buzz of cicadas, I could see the guests mingling inside. Dr. Sherman Flowers, cornered by J. Puckett Middlebrooks, the gregarious Flint gynecologist, had a wild, scared look of a squirrel in a brush fire. Lee Bob Parker, Karl Wright's son-in-law, stood in a circle of men and brayed laughter. I wondered where his notorious wife was.

I felt the pressure of a long fingernail starting at my neck and running down from my shoulder blades to the small of my back. I reached behind me, patting a hip I thought was Shelley's. "Scratch my back and I'll follow you anywhere," I said. "In fact, you don't even have to scratch my back." The hip moved closer and I felt the pressure of an abdomen more ample than Shelley's against my buttocks, of breasts more buxom against my back. "That's very reassuring," said a voice rich as the mint syrup in a julep.

"Oops," I said, turning to make the acquaintance of Beulah Parker, who didn't back up an inch to give me room to turn around.

"You're the new doctor," she observed. Her eyes sparkled like her diamond earrings and necklace. "Welcome to Grady."

"I've been here for a while."

"But now it looks like you're going to stay."

"Do you know something I don't."

"Probably." From Shelley, I'd gathered that Beulah was over forty. She was either well-preserved or cosmetically overhauled, maybe both. Her black evening gown plunged nearly to her navel, and I was having trouble looking her in the eyes. "Come with me. I want to show you something before you meet Daddy."

"I've ordered drinks."

"They won't run out of spirits before you swing back by."

She led me through the happy conglomeration of beautiful people, doctors and their ornamental wives, well scrubbed, well dressed, well decorated, well healed--a far cry from the farmers and mill workers I'd been rubbing elbows with at Trafford Memorial Hospital. As we passed back into the house and entered the thick oak door of the library, I glanced at Shelly. She was chatting with Dr. "Country" Trulane, a distinguished ophthalmologist in a tweed jacket. She watched us over his shoulder, her tongue making a lump in her cheek.

The library walls were lined with Moroccan bound volumes I got the feeling had never been read. There was a zebra skin on the heart pine floor and a cape buffalo above a baroque mantle, but the most extraordinary thing was a shoulder mount of a giraffe. From its towering nine-foot neck, sad brown eyes gazed from the ten-foot ceilings.

Beulah noticed my perverse attraction. "You really want to piss off a lot of bleeding hearts," she said, "shoot a giraffe."

"Did you shoot it?"

"No, Lee Bob did. Daddy took us on safari. Daddy shot the buffalo, and Lee Bob bagged the giraffe."

"What did you kill?" I'd never imagined anybody shooting a giraffe. In fact, it had never occurred to me to hunt anything at all, although I'd trapped some mice in my time.

"Crocodiles. I dressed in a pith helmet, suntans, and gauze; broke the heart of the great white hunter, an English chap; and I shot crocodiles."

"What was that like?"

"The crocs or the bwana?" she winked. "There wasn't much to the crocodiles. About like shooting alligators or turtles. The rifle makes a big boom and a waterspout. They thrash around and sink. Sometimes they wallow up on shore and die. The bwanas wallow up."

I couldn't believe I was having this conversation. "What do you, uh, do with a dead giraffe. Can you eat them?"

"The meat's musty, I'm told. We fed it to the crocs."

"Except the head and shoulders, which is a considerable percentage of your giraffe."

"Well, the boys skinned it and decapitated it. The crocs got the rest. Then we shot some crocs."

"The *boys*?"

"Yes," she smiled, "the boys. There are no girl porters in Africa."

"Didn't the boys want any giraffe meat?"

"We gave them the buff."

"Then you shot some boys?"

"No."

"Well, tell me, when you shoot a giraffe, do you have to jump back quickly and yell *timberrrr*! or do they just sort of collapse in one spot."

Beulah reached for my cummerbund, pulling me forward, smiling, pretending that my shirt needed tucking in. I felt the scratch of her fingernails. "They do a lot of falling," she said, wetting her upper lip with her tongue. "But the giraffe isn't what I brought you in here to show you. Try not to be such a smart ass."

There was a pregnant silence until suddenly I felt the gaze of another pair of eyes, besides the giraffe's and the cape buffalo's. "Well, what then?" Shelly said. "What do you want to show the smart ass besides your giraffe?" She was leaning in the doorway, holding the stem of an empty champagne glass.

"Shelly!" I said.

Beulah still held my belt buckle. A diamond scratched my belly. She smiled, unabashed, amused. Her shadowed eyelids lowered. "Well, Shelly, won't you join us. I have something that will interest you, too."

"You've got something by the belt buckle that *used* to interest me," Shelly said, leaving and closing the door behind her.

"Shelly, wait!" I felt my face flush.

"Don't worry about Shelly," smiled Beulah. "We're ancient adversaries. Come over here." She would have pulled me by the belt buckle if I'd let her, but I lifted her hand from the front of my trousers and followed her to a framed map that bristled with colorful push pins adjacent to tiny triangular flags. I was anxious to find Shelly and get away from these festivities, from this place, away from Beulah's dangerous magnetism. I hoped Shelly had not already left me.

The map, which depicted Georgia and portions of Alabama and Florida, looked like a campaign plan for a military invasion. All the miniature flags were labeled. Lilies of the Valley and Southern Vision were two names I recognized. Also identified were several regional hospitals, medical and dental offices, a chiropractor or two. The cluster of pennants and push pins was densest in the southwest portion of Georgia, south of Macon, west of I-75, and north of the Florida line, although a few pins and pennants sprinkled over into Florida's panhandle and across the Chattahoochee River into southeast Alabama.

"The blue pins Daddy controls. The red ones he wants to acquire."

"What's he do with the blue ones? It looks like he's trying to sew up the health industry in these parts." I was nervous. Shelly says I sound like a Hollywood cowboy when I fake a southern accent.

"He makes money. The doctors that work at the blue ones do very well."

"Like Country Trulane?"

"He could serve as a representative example."

"Your father wants a regional monopoly."

"We like to call it a *private for-profit comprehensive health care system*. I wanted you to see it in case Daddy offers you something."

"I don't plan on being around long enough do anything speculative, but I can't help noticing there's a red pin in Trafford Memorial. And one in Putnam Memorial in Flint."

Beulah's eyebrows went up. She smiled, removing a Grady County pin next to the Trafford pennant. "That's a mistake," she said. "That doesn't belong there." She fixed the pin into my lapel and patted it. She averted her chin and fixed my eyes in hers. Her heavy floral perfume radiated from her white neck and deep cleavage. I felt like I was standing up to my waist in a patch of honeysuckle, and I knew I'd better run. Southern women have a softness around the edges that's dangerous to poor Yankee boys unschooled in seduction in sultry climates. The scorpion hearts within these oh, so alabaster breasts. The Confederates would have won if they'd turned things over to their ladies.

The whole scene was feudal, Karl Wright standing ready to parcel our territory and medical facilities for loyalty to his cause.

I broke away from her gaze, and her cool hand moved from my lapel to the side of my neck. "I better, uh, mosey down the trail."

If Beulah was moved by my hasty departure, she didn't show it. She seated herself on the top of an enormous mahogany desk, the hem of her sequined dress rising halfway up her thighs. "We'll be in touch," she said with a slow reptilian smile.

Shelly was waiting, seated in a wingback chair, thoughtfully nibbling her lower lip, her beeper still clipped into the neckline of her dress. She was smiling. And she looked very beautiful to me, although I admit some of the romantic spontaneity of the moment may have been chemically induced by Beulah. Shelly and Beulah represented opposite notions of apollonian and dionysian beauty. Shelly's features were classical, streamlined, functional, while Beulah's body was fecund, luxurious, and seductive. Of course, the objectivity of my analysis was not to be entirely trusted, since I was in love with Shelly and Beulah had just finished fizzing my blood like ginger ale.

"You ready to go?" I said, halfway expecting Shelly to be angry.

She smiled, "Have you seen enough of Beulah's trophies to decide whether you want to be one of them?"

"I'll throw in with you," I said.

We found our host, Carl Wright, and paid our respects. Like nearly every other man present, including the servants, he wore a tux. We shook hands and he looked me up and down, maybe admiring the eclectic nature of my outfit. His handshake was firm, but cool like Beulah's fingers. He was a solidly built man in his early seventies with a shock of silver hair and eyes like brass. He smiled absently, letting his gaze settle on Shelly. "Don't be surprised if you hear from me in a month or so," he warned, ushering us to the door.

"Where'd you get the red pin?" Shelly asked.

Chapter Four

The first time Shelly and I'd made love was two months ago in early February, a week after Dr. Hogue had his first heart attack. I'd hospitalized Hogue and witnessed an incarnation of the adage that doctors make the worst patients, especially when they are hung over. Dr. Hogue was going to survive, but he was going to have to slow down considerably.

Shelly and I were on call together. In those days it made sense to coordinate our shifts because I didn't have a car and we could use the ambulance for emergencies or just to ride around so long as we stayed within range of the radio and within the boundaries of Grady County. Our courtship involved interminable hours of gin rummy, study sessions with my medical journals and her law books, and dogeared, perennial jokes. "What's the difference between a catfish and a lawyer?" I asked.

"I don't know."

"One's a scum-sucking bottom dweller. The other is a fish."

"What's more dangerous than a drunk turpentiner in a pulpwood truck?"

"What?"

"A doctor in a Cessna."

"No, I mean what's a turpentiner?"

"You need to go back *home*, Stone."

I'd realized from first sight that the blond paramedic with the boyish haircut, who unsuccessfully disguised her sexuality in maroon polyester trousers and a white shirt with epaulets, was one of the prettiest women I'd ever seen, but I had no intention of staying at Trafford a moment longer than necessary to pay off the repair bill on my car, and Shelly, I'd found, was no easy sexual acquisition. Besides, I was involved in a long distance romance with a Miami nurse--who, I eventually realized, had been working on a MRS.MD. degree and who wanted to pursue her studies at Jackson Memorial in Miami rather than correspondent course work. "My main squeeze wrote that she thought it best that we stop writing," I confessed in the ER one Saturday night.

"You don't sound shattered," Shelly replied, licking the lead of her pencil and making a note in a margin.

"Well, maybe she's just not a talented writer, but lately her letters seem to be taking a census of my personal tastes and politics. She wants to know if I like French provincial furniture and Yorkshire terriers. She wonders if we'll vacation in Highlands, North Carolina, or Hilton Head; if I'll prefer golf to tennis. I mean, people in love don't have to catalogue all that, do they? It was like she was taking a course under me."

"*Under* you!" exclaimed Shelly. "Isn't this tart even liberated? You're lucky to be shed of her, Stone. Take my advice and find you a nice little Southern girl with nymphomaniacal attitudes towards sex and lesions on her fallopian tubes, somebody who wouldn't be caught dead married to a doctor, but who might condescend to sleeping with one on the sly. That's what you need to get through your tour in Dixie."

"How about you?"

"My fallopian tubes are quite intact, thank you."

"Do you have any of the remaining aforementioned qualifications?" I asked.

She thought for a moment. "Well, I wouldn't be caught dead married to a doctor."

Late that night, after I finished my duties at the hospital, she drove me home and stayed until morning.

Thus Shelly and I began as colleagues, then progressed from friendship to love in a small country town where everyone knew what we were up to but where most wished us well. We paid tribute to Southern respectability by keeping separate quarters, although we became all but inseparable during our limited leisure, and on the night of Saturday, February 6, 1983 (according to my notebook), Shelly left her ambulance, replete with blue Star of Life, parked overnight in my front yard for everyone who happened by to see and conclude that no fresh tire prints led to the emergency vehicle covered with hoar frost. *Shelly! Oh, Shelly!* the February 5 entry laconically concludes, beneath the procedural notes of February 4 concerning Leroy Easter's polyps and Eddie Oglesbee's gout, which hurt so bad, he testified, he couldn't shine a flashlight on it.

Shelly and I both awoke before dawn--after love, content and hopeful about the future, our lungs full of clean air. The solid pine of my rented farmhouse creaked as the temperature dropped just before sunrise. We were huddled together in my brass bed which, like most of my other belongings, had been provided by my landlords Commissioner Worthy and his wife Miss Ida, who'd proved the most formidable adversary to my attempts at leaving Grady. No service, credit, or privilege was extended to me without her approval. I even suspected her of screening my mail.

I brushed back Shelly's bangs. "What's a nice sexy girl like you doing riding country roads in a meat wagon? Tell me the absolute truth. An EMT! Such a mighty ghoulish profession for a cheerleader type with a B.A. in English and philosophy."

"I'm bloodthirsty," she said. I knew that Shelly had been in college at UNC at Chapel Hill when her parents were both killed in an automobile accident with a logging truck. This knowledge rendered her jokes about dangerous doctors and drunk drivers dark and personal. There had been just enough insurance for her

18

to finish her bachelors but not enough for law school, so she'd returned to Grady, where she owned her parents' house. She had planned to save her money, go to law school at Vanderbilt, and become a storefront and civil rights lawyer defending society's less fortunate.

Well, most of it made sense, sort of. English was a good pre-law major, and philosophy went along with English, paving the way for the predominantly idealistic motives of students in the America of the late 70's, to become instruments of positive social change. Tah dah. All of us were idealistic, most of us were messianic. My sister Nancy, one example, became a social worker, married my med-school roommate at Stanford, Jim Maloy, and hauled him off to a mission hospital in Guatemala, where she gratified post-adolescent fantasies of joining the Peace Corps. Half of my graduating class expressed at one time or another desires to serve stints in jungle tuberculosis sanitariums and leper colonies.

Not me. I wanted to save mankind from the ivory towers and hallowed halls of academic medicine, and I was not at all opposed to a clean shirt while doing it. How ironic that I, perhaps more than my other friends, had become inadvertently indentured to mankind. I didn't think Shelly was ever going to make it as a lawyer, although she had the brains and the determination to become one. She had deeply rooted notions of right and wrong. She pictured herself dispatching slumlords, saving endangered animals, and crusading for civil liberties, but I knew she'd make a terrible attorney if she were hired to champion a cause she didn't believe in. Most lawyers I knew had developed a pragmatic and floating ethical system to survive. Shelly wasn't morally flexible. Nor was she going to be able to submit to and embrace a system of law whose most powerful advocates were male. She was a woman of action not abstraction, and everybody seemed to know that but Shelly.

She took my stethoscope from the pocket of my lab coat and listened to my heart as she slid her hand under the covers and rested it about four inches beneath my navel. "I want to see if you love me," she explained.

"Oh? Well, why?" I wiggled away from her, needing rest. She rolled over, hemming me up at the edge of the bed. "That's cold," I said.

"Why what?" She removed the stethoscope from her ears and hooked it around her neck.

"Why do you drive an ambulance?"

"Right now? You really want to know right now why I drive an ambulance?"

"Yes, right now. I want to know right now. This is something I must know."

She smiled, rolling over to her stomach and resting her chin on a pillow. Her smile dissolved. "When my parents were killed in 1976," she said, "ambulance service was provided by Hooks and Stokes funeral homes. Like nearly everything else, the services were segregated. If you were white and needed an ambulance, you called Hooks. If you were black you called Stokes. The drivers were assistant morticians or flunkies, who believed that speeding to the hospital was the best way to save victims' lives."

"Talk about a conflict of interest!"

Shelly smiled. "Yes, the mortuary got a hundred dollars if you lived and several thousand if you died, but Hooks and Stokes did the best they could until Dr. Hogue persuaded Robert McCormick Jones to buy the county an ambulance." She threw a leg over my hip.

"Is that *the* Jones of Coca Cola fame, the owner of Toa Plantation?"

Jones had a philanthropic interest in Grady County. He'd bought quinine and hired a public health nurse to treat malaria back in 1936.

"Has anybody asked him to donate money to Trafford?" The pitch of my voice changed, and my breathing had deepened.

"Not his style. He gives seed money to non-profit charitable ventures only, or his foundation does--brick and mortar stuff, not day-to-day operating expenses."

"Well, Trafford has non-profit status, in reality if not in charter." I took her hand. Trafford was waterlogged by debt, about to go under for the third time.

"Anyway, the county got an ambulance," she went on. "Dr. Hogue sent his son Buster to paramedic school at Flint Junior College. He flunked out, and Dr. Carl offered to send me."

I think I was passing Shelly's love test. My pulse was making tambourines out of my tympana, but I continued our chat, playing it cool. "Why you?"

"He figured I was a good bet. I'm a good student, so he knew I wouldn't have much trouble finishing the program, and he knew I'd be around for at least the four or five years it would take me to save enough for law school. He knew I wouldn't be tempted elsewhere because I could live rent free in the house my parents left me. I think he also hoped I'd be a good influence on Buster, maybe marry him."

"Buster! No wonder he has daggers in his eyes when I'm around."

"Not daggers, he just pouts a little. Buster's sweet. He's having a little trouble living up to daddy's expectations."

"Like hauling you to the altar."

She smiled. "Well, that wasn't part of my plan, but driving an ambulance appealed to me. On the practical side, the long on-duty hours with nothing to do give me plenty of time for my studies. On the ideological front, I was ready to move away from philosophical abstraction into a real world of action."

"I act, therefore I am?"

"Analysis breeds paralysis."

"Did the death of your parents have anything to do with it?" I asked this hesitantly, wondering if I broached a subject too personal. It's hard not to get personal when I'm naked.

"There was probably an unconscious drive, yes. A paramedic could have saved my parents, at least my mother. So I became a paramedic to bring them back symbolically? Hum, you're very bright, Stone. You're wrong, but you're very bright, and you'd make a marvelous psychologist, but it was the *golden hour* that converted me."

Simply put, the "golden hour" was the 60-minute time frame recognized in Vietnam. For about one hour the human body can withstand severe hypotensive shock. After an hour of very low blood pressure, irreversible organ failure sets in--brain death, kidney failure. Extreme trauma victims die if they aren't stabilized before they arrive at a hospital.

"My mother was thrown clear of the car, and Daddy was pinned inside. When Hooks' ambulance finally got there, the driver tried unsuccessfully for thirty or forty minutes to extricate Daddy before taking Mamma to the hospital. She died, of shock mostly, before they could get there." Shelly had pulled the cover under her chin. She was smiling faintly, staring at the olive morning light beyond the window. "I don't know if a modern 911 ambulance system with a Jaws of Life and a trained paramedic could have saved Daddy, but I know Mamma didn't have to die."

We were silent for a few moments. Then the birds started with the peeping of chickadees and the throaty warble of a wren. From the far side of Loonie Lake we heard an owl call. "My parents," she continued, "had almost nothing in common except love and me, yet they almost never fought. They didn't even go to the same church. I buried Mamma and cremated Daddy. His ashes are on my mantel at home."

"Shelly," I said playfully, pressing the button of her nose, "I love you."

She smiled. "I know, and we have one golden hour before our love life shuts down and we have to start getting ready to go back to work saving lives and fighting windmills," she said, throwing off the covers. She swung herself up, straddling my stomach, arching her back, and starting up with the stethoscope again. I looked up to see her face centered over her rosy tipped breasts that hardened in the brisk morning air. She placed the stethoscope on my chest, rolling her eyes upward then laughing. "God Stone, I think you're going to infarct!"

I held her waist, resting my thumbs against the arch of her rib cage. She removed the stethoscope and dropped it to the floor, easing backwards until I entered her. We made slow thoughtful love, and afterwards, lying on our sides, facing each other, I held her waist again, just above a high thin hip, and marveled how my fingers could nearly touch behind her back, and I realized at that moment what most young men take for granted--the exquisite, tingling beauty of being in love at daybreak with a strong lovely woman. Reaching for the stethoscope, she put the earpieces into her ears and listened to her own heart. "Too bad, Stone, I'm not in love with you yet."

"Here, let me listen!"

"Nothing doing, I'd never seek a man's council concerning problems of the heart. I'd never use a male midwife, psychic, or gynecologist. Take it from me, I'm not in love with you yet." She hesitated. "But you can keep trying. I think you're starting to soften me up."

Chapter Five
(11 April 1983 Trafford Hospital)

It took ten days for Hackamore Singletree to contract serum sickness, an immune reaction to antivenin. He arrived at Trafford at daybreak and was waiting for me when I got there. He had, in his own words, *took ugly*. His face was the shape of a catcher's mitt, eyelids swollen like lemons, his hands like boxing gloves.

I led him into an office and examined his thumb and ankle, where necrotic skin had started to slough and stink, but which were starting to heal. Snakebite kills the surrounding flesh and causes decay. Hack wasn't going to lose much thumb, but the ankle bite would leave a nice dent. The massive doses of antivenin had minimized tissue damage. I changed his dressings, gave him injections of steroids and penicillin, and wrote a prescription.

He grinned like a jack-o-lantern. "You can say what you want about Hartwell the vet, but he never left me looking like this."

"You better stay home for a couple of days."

"I can't. I got bush hooks out and trotlines." Bush hooks were fishing lines tied to tree branches. Trotlines were fishing lines tied at intervals to a long single line submerged in a creek or river.

"Let Frog run them."

"Haw! I'd just as soon give Frog a key to my deep freezer as tell him where my bush hooks and lines are at. Something's robbing my catfish as it is."

"Raccoons and alligators," I speculated, "turtles."

"Something else, too."

"How do you know?"

"Tracks."

I raised my eyebrows. "The Gatorman?"

"Something."

"Something with a wide foot and claws?"

"There you go."

"I sure would like to see those tracks."

"Go on down there and hunt you up a set."

"Would you guide me down there."

"You'd be worse than Frog on my catfish. Yankees ain't got much sense of propriety. Didn't you read about what Sherman did to Atlanta when he passed through?"

"You ought to see what the Yankees have done to Florida. Will you take me into the Toa?"

"What for?"

"Because I pumped fifteen hundred dollars worth of antivenin into you and saved your ass from dying of snake bite."

Hack grinned like a tear in a medicine ball. "My ass looks like a lot of things right now," he said, "and *saved* ain't one of them."

I ordered him to take his pills and come back in the following Saturday, my afternoon off. I didn't believe the Gatorman hype, but if Hack was well enough, we'd visit the Swamp of Toa, the vast wetland I'd wanted to see since I'd read about it in the *Smithsonian*. Its singular beauty derived from the fact that this section of Georgia's costal plains was honeycombed with artesian wells and underground streams, boasting three aquifers. While in Miami, I'd driven over to the Everglades National Park and viewed the seemingly endless marshes from wooden platform and walkways, but I'd never seen a true cyprus and tupelo swamp, and I was anxious to visit one before I returned to civilization and was called upon to describe south Georgia at cocktail parties.

By the time Hack had left, the waiting room was filling up as usual with impoverished locals with toothaches, chest pain, impacted bowels, head lice, ring worms, ingrown toenails, and broken bones. Whenever I went to work it was as though I had stepped back into a history of maladies I'd thought obsolete in this era of modern medicine, the 1980's. Patients arrived wearing homespun poultices, plasters, and sachets. They reeked of their own tinctures, ointments, and salves. Dr. Hogue walked among them like a fatigued general through a battlefield, snapping orders to his adjutant Nurse Holt, culling the seriously wounded, sending the others along, assigning the disagreeable and hypochondriac illnesses to me. I'd become a specialist in head colds and gonorrhea among other things. We peeked in eyes, examined tongues, and poked lymph nodes with our index fingers, organizing the critical, the chronic, the psychosomatic, the expectant, the terminal. Babies squalled, children skirmished, the elderly moaned. Trafford's waiting room looked like an anteroom to hell.

At 9:30 a profound hush came over the waiting room, stilling even the extraordinary Dr. Hogue. The obese white woman whose tympanic membrane I inspected snatched her ear away, yanking her head toward the door. At the entrance an ancient black woman, powerful and serene, stood solidly in her walker, her nappy hair haloed in a shaft of morning light. The wide old woman remained silent in an aura of profound monolithic dignity until the great-granddaughter at her side spoke quietly: "Big Mamma want to see the new doctor."

Dr. Hogue himself stood stunned, his baggy head cocked to one side. There was a thick and palpable stillness. Not a whine, sniffle, or cough from the patients. Their heads swung magnetically toward Big Mamma, their jaws agape. I stepped forward timidly, awed like the motley others. "What's wrong with her?" I said.

"Nothin' ain't wrong," the girl answered. "She Miss Ethel Hargrove. My name Cyrilla. Big Mamma just want to see the new doctor."

I extended my hand as Miss Ethel's hazel eyes *studied* me, the only word to describe that scrutiny. Her deeply lined face was the dark golden brown of tupelo honey. She took my hand but didn't shake it. She held it in both her hands, unsupported by the walker as she watched my face. Then she placed the palm of one hand on my chest, pursing her lips, still perusing my eyes. Finally, she turned, leaving in fluid and mechanical combinations as she advanced with the walker. She passed Dr. Hogue, her eyes dead ahead. "He'll do," she told him.

"What?" He tugged his ear lobe, jutting his lower teeth.

"He'll do aw right."

Chapter Six

I followed Hack down the logging road into the Swamp of Toa, until a plant he called a "whoa vine" stopped me dead in my tracks. "Yow! Ouch!" The vine was thick as a pencil with black-tipped thorns, one of which was embedded to the hilt just above my knee. Hack had recovered from his serum sickness, but not before he had taken full and perverse advantage of his monstrous visage, appearing from behind gallberry bushes, grunting and waving his arms at fishermen who knocked over their five gallon buckets and dropped their cane poles. By the end of the week he'd fanned the fires of the Gatorman legend and caused a proliferation of reported sightings, so many that Hack's sidekick Sheriff Rooster Bootman threatened to lock him up for disturbing the peace.

"Watch where you're going, Doc."

"I was watching. I was looking for snakes." I pulled down my trousers and examined the purple puncture.

"You let me watch for snakes," he grinned, holding up his thumb. "I'm an expert. Look *down*. The poison ones can't climb."

The logging road became a path, then disappeared among palmettos, gallberries, and loblolly pine. The only trails now were game trails and our own watery footprints in the rich, black mud. We entered the bottom, where the thick canopy of the bigbellied cypress and bay trees blocked off the sunlight, choking out underbrush and making the walking easier. Before I'd come to Grady, I wouldn't have known a sycamore from a blackjack oak. But I had begun keeping a notebook, which served as a fieldbook for cultural and natural history. As soon as Hack discovered my neophyte interest in wildlife, he readily supplied information. He showed me my first living specimen of poison ivy, for example, as soon as we got out of the truck, and another fascinating plant with sticky stem and small pink flowers. When Hack touched the feathery leaves they folded up, withdrawing from tactile stimulation.

"That thing has a brain!" I exclaimed.

"*Mimosa pudica*," said Hack as I sketched and scribbled in my notebook.

From that first excursion into the Toa, Hack began taking a curious responsibility for my innocence, my ignorance of anything outside the city limits of a northern metropolis. Shelly provided an indispensable bridge between my textbook naivete and the folk wisdom of my patients, but Hack was to provide a cornucopia of swamp and woodland lore to which I would eventually become a willing acolyte. Still, I wasn't mentally prepared for an actual field trip into a wilderness replete with snakes, alligators, and bloodthirsty mosquitoes, "swamp angels" Hack called them. I guess I expected the same kind of elevated wooden walkways that provided access to the Everglades. As soon as we stepped into the boggy gloom of the Toa, I became ill at ease.

"Isn't there a better way to get there?"

"Get where?"

"Wherever we're going."

"Well, there's a easier way. We could have driven fifty miles around the swamp and gone in from Mulgrove Ridge, but that way you'd miss seeing the flora and fauna of this neck of the woods. A case in point is that gentleman laying over yonder."

Until then I had thought over yonder was a vague area more or less near the horizon, but just ahead in thick coils was a dusky snake, its triangular head raised. "Jesus!" Every muscle in my body contracted as though connected by a common nerve, and my skin tightened into gooseflesh. "God!"

The baleful head tracked Hack, who eased up beside the reptile, not three feet away. The moccasin yawned, showing the wide white interior of its mouth. "He's warning us," said Hack. "That's why he's called a cottonmouth."

"Shoot him," I advised, noticing with alarm that Hack's revolver was still holstered.

"What for?" he said. "They ain't fit to eat, and they keep the Yankees out of the swamp." He grinned. "At least they did up to now. Anyway, what's Miss Shelly gone say if I murder off one of God's little creatures?" He squatted before the reptile and took off his Stetson, waiting for the snake to close its mouth. The black tongue flipped out, and the neck cocked, tracking the hat, which Hack slowly moved back and forth in front of his knees.

"What are you doing?" I said.

"Shhhhh."

"You get bit again, you're too heavy for me to carry out of here."

"Hush," said Hack. He waited until the snake stopped tracking. It lowered its head and had begun crawling away when Hack covered its head with the hat brim, pinning the head gently and carefully grasping the snake's neck. Then, supporting the thick body with his other hand, he lifted it and brought it to the spot where I was struggling to control my knees and bladder.

"*Akistron, piciverous, pisciverous,*" he smiled. "Eastern cottonmouth water moccasin. Come over here. I'm gone show you something. See that hole between his eye and his nostril? That's why he's called a pit viper. It's a heat sensor, infrared. All your poisonous snakes around here have that pit and this here elliptical pupil like the one you see in this gentleman's eye. Cat eyed."

Locals claimed the cottonmouth can't bite underwater without drowning. I asked Hack about it.

"Well Doc, like the name '*pisciverous*' implies, they eat fish. Look here." Shifting his grip behind the snake's jaws, he opened its mouth with the fingernail of his middle finger and pointed out the curved hypodermic fangs. "Right here's the poison glands." He tickled a puffy jaw and a drop of amber liquid beaded at the tip of the hollow, fishbone fang.

"It's easy to see how you get snakebit," I said. By this time I'd forgotten my fear of snakes and had become absorbed in Hack's encyclopedic chit-chat. It still gave me a mild shock every time I heard specialized vocabulary garbled by a mouth full of tobacco juice or grits, a prejudice I had brought down with me from Washington. My association with Hack was rapidly dispelling the theory that backwoods Southerners were ignorant.

"You ever wonder how a snake can swallow a rabbit whole without suffocating? Well, he can open up his mouth wide as the biggest part of his body. He uses that little windpipe there that runs up under his tongue to breath when he's got a throat full. Have you got a good look, Doc? You need a good look at that windpipe." Suddenly, he squeezed the snake's jaws and squirted twin jets of fluid on my shirt front and trousers.

I stumbled backward and sat down hard, splattering mud outward from the seat of my breaches, furious. The snake didn't appreciate Hack's joke any more than I did. It lashed and hissed, struggling, it seemed, more to bite Hack than to escape. Hack, laughing uproariously, tried to untangle himself from the writhing body and lashing tail to throw the snake down. Horrified and furious, I watched the big man hold the snake at arm's length, drop it, and step backward. The angry cottonmouth reared the front third of its body length and began striking. Hack laughed and danced in his heavy boots, avoiding the fangs, holding his sides until he sat down in the mud beside me, teary-eyed from laughter. The snake slid noiselessly into the water and glided away, its body riding high on the surface.

"That was the d-dumbest d-damned trick I've ever seen in my life," I stammered. I was ready to kill him. Righteous indignation mixed with shame for being afraid.

"Don't be mad, Doc. Here, have a drink." He produced a flask from his canvas jacket, politely wiping the neck with his palm before offering it. I glared at him. "Come on Doc, be a sport," he grinned.

I took a half-hearted sip from the bottle. Immediately the fumes entered my nostrils and watered my eyes. The liquid burned a raw trail down my esophagus as I swallowed and coughed. My anger flared again, but I knew Hack's offer of moonshine whiskey was not a practical joke.

"Hold it in your mouth a little longer," he said. "The saliva will help it down."

We passed the bottle back and forth several times, and I started feeling better almost immediately. Strangely drugged with adrenaline and 130 proof firewater,

I discovered a sudden beauty in the swamp around us. The afternoon sunlight broke through the dense canopy into the lush green of mossy banks that contained the meandering dark water. The Gothic bay roots and stalagmite cypress knees, which Hack had taught me were the breathing apparatus for the broad-based trees, rose above the onyx water, reflected perfectly as on a chrome surface. Bright yellow cabbage butterflies mimicked their twins in the water. And the cacophony of swamp sounds became melodious in the muted light. The mosquitoes hummed and the molecular waterbugs worried the water. For the first time in my life, I had an inkling of a transcendental poet's communion with nature. If I ever got out of Grady, I knew I'd remember the early spring field trip into the Toa with this strange, rough man.

"We better get moving," he said. "We're going to be after dark getting out of here as it is."

Chapter Seven

I followed for another hour along the banks of a labyrinthine blackwater stream Hack called Little Sowbelly Branch. Suddenly he stopped, and I bumped into him. I was used to his pausing to point out potential entries for my notebook, which in a single afternoon had become filled with rough drawings of animal tracks and plants reputed to have medicinal value. After the snake episode I guess I was following close.

We were at the intersection of two deer trails. Several sets of sharply pointed cloven doe tracks pocked the area; among them was a set of larger prints with wider clefts and dewclaw impressions, probably characteristics of a buck. Other animal tracks I now recognized as raccoon laced the dark mud near the branch.

"What you make of that, Doc?" Hack said, pointing to deep impressions in the mud."What do *you* reckon made those tracks?"

"A bear?" Although the track itself was slightly longer than wide, there were distinct claw-marks four or five inches long.

"It's too long for a bear," Hack said.

"What then?"

Whatever it was, it had come and gone more than once, dragging something through the mud, something that had blurred some of the prints like an alligator dragging its tail, or a beaver. Whatever it was, it didn't follow so precise a trail as the deer, which tend to stick to the same path. This thing had moved back and forth in the same general direction.

"Why doesn't it follow a trail?" I asked Hack. "Why does it wander around?"

"Predators wander around. And animals that walk upright," he said. "An animal walking on its hind feet can see over the palmettoes and make for a *general* direction."

"What walks on its hind legs besides a man?"

"Nothing I know of."

"A bear? Are there bears in the swamp?"

"Yeah, they're a few bears in here, and they stand on their hind legs every now and again, but they get around on all fours. These tracks are from one two-legged animal that looks to weigh about three-fifty to four-hundred pounds, judging by how deep he's sinking down."

"Come on, Hack. Those footprints aren't any deeper than yours, and you weigh what? 250?" I had already anthropomorphically labeled the tracks "footprints," but I still couldn't believe whatever left them was human.

"My feet ain't that wide. This thing's bigger than me unless it's carrying a hundred pounds besides the twenty or thirty it's dragging."

"Could that be a tail?"

Hack grinned. "I reckon it could be. You ever known a man to drag a tail, Doc?"

"What makes you think it's a man?"

"Well, I guess it *could* be a woman, but she'd be a *big* old gal."

"What makes you think it's human? I'm no woodsman, but medical training tells me those tracks aren't your everyday humanoid footprints. Just look at the length of those toenails."

"Well, it ain't no animal I've ever seen, unless it's a kangaroo, and there didn't used to be no kangaroos in the Toa."

"How tall is it?"

"I wouldn't know about that."

Hack decided to take a drink and think about it. He produced his flask and I joined him. I was more than a little concerned that we were in the Toa with a three-hundred-and-fifty-pound creature that hadn't been classified in the annals of natural history, compounded by the fact that it was getting dark.

Hack knelt beside the trail and pondered one of the clearer prints for a long time. "Well, I thought it might be somebody wearing something on his feet, maybe with his feet wrapped up, but it ain't. He's barefoot, and he's a flat-footed sumbitch, too."

"What kind of man would walk barefoot in the middle of Toa Swamp?" I still didn't believe the footprints were human.

"Somebody who ain't got no shoes?" he smiled. "Thom McCann don't make shoes to fit a foot like that."

"And you think these tracks were made by what people have been calling the *Gatorman*."

"I sure do." He scratched his whiskers, mostly white but peppered with black and red. "At least they were made by what *some* people call the Gatorman. Doc, squat down here and take a whiff and tell me what you smell besides a stinking flat-footed critter," he laughed. "Come on. I ain't kidding."

I lowered myself to my hands and knees and sniffed the track. There was a distinct odor, vaguely familiar, but I couldn't quite place it. "I've smelled that odor before," I told Hack, "but I can't quite remember where. Maybe it will come to me later."

"Well, it ain't something *I've* smelled before."

Chapter Eight

When Hack dropped me off at Shelly's house, he barely came to a complete stop. Shelly was, as he'd predicted she would be, "mad enough to bite a polecat." I crept inside. She was washing dishes, which was not a good sign since I'd been invited for dinner.

She gave me the once-over, quickly surmising that I'd been drinking. She was washing the dishes like soldiers on KP, knocking the food off by banging them together. I stood first on one foot, then the other, hoping stupidly for a transformation of mood.

"Well, let's see," she said. "We have evolved to the point of our relationship when you want to come staggering in with muddy boots after dark, expecting your supper, after having been out drinking moonshine all day with your redneck friends. Am I right?"

"Shelly, wait till I tell you what we found!"

"Let me guess." She raised her eyebrows. "You went off into the wilderness with a hairy prophet and discovered the maleness twentieth century technology robbed from you. You've come to terms with your testosterone."

"Shelly . . . ." I shifted my weight from one foot to the other, afraid to sit down.

"You and the Neanderthal stripped down to face paint and loincloth and danced around a campfire, screaming yourselves into touch with your primal past. A necessary stage in your transition to Good Old Boy."

"Shelly, we found the Gatorman's footprints."

She made a perfect circle of her mouth, arching her eyebrows. "Oh, well excuse me for being a little piqued. I thought you stood me up, let me fix your supper, and made me worry about you, for some trifle. I didn't know that you were on an important assignment, out solving the mysteries of the supernatural. Why didn't you tell me what you and your acromegalic friend were up to? You discovered the footprints of the swamp monster children and drunks are talking about." Shelly's fist was on her hip, clenching a red checkered dishtowel.

"You can't make me mad, Shelly," I said, getting mad.

"Yes, I can. I can make you mad as hell." She shook the dishtowel in my face, a banner of contempt.

"Look, I need to eat something. I'm a little drunk, and I need to put something in my stomach." I was tired and dizzy and I wanted to sit down at the kitchen table, but I didn't want her taller than me. I didn't think she would clobber me with a pan or stab me with a knife, but towering over me would give her a psychological advantage.

"Oh, is the poor thing a little drunk? He's been out all afternoon crusading and chasing the jabberwock and now he's a little drunk and needs something in his tummy. Well, just give me a second or two so I can whip something up to take the place of the crab meat souffle I fed to Clarice."

Clarice was Shelly's bluetick hound. Hearing her name spoken with such acidity, Clarice uncurled from beneath the table and padded mournfully out of the harm she sensed was brewing. She was an old dog and wise, of flappy dugs and innumerable litters. I realized that Shelly had the psychological advantage, whether I sat down or not.

"There were wide footprints with long claws," I said defensively. "They led to the part of the swamp Hack calls the Capachequi, the hills in the 'swampy province' described in De Soto's chronicles."

"Well, isn't it marvelous that you were able to locate the monster's footprints so quickly? I mean, I'll bet you two nimrods practically went straight to the creature's tracks, didn't you." Her cropped butterscotch head nodded. Her eyes were bright with anger. "That's pretty good, the Toa being some sixty-thousand acres. You two were pretty lucky to just stumble onto the creature like that."

"What are you saying?"

"I'm saying that you look foolish enough around here without letting Hack Singletree make a laughingstock out of the new boy in town. That clodhopper went into the swamp this morning and made those tracks to set you up."

"Hack was at school this morning. I called him there."

"Well, he did it yesterday then," she said, slamming a dish into the cabinet. "Anyway, school's out."

"Hack wouldn't do that. He doesn't have the time or inclination to do something like that." I walked into the living room and lay down on the couch. Maybe a submissive gesture would disarm Shelly. She followed me into the living room with a fist full of silver utensils. "Get up from there," she ordered. Then she returned to the kitchen and threw the silverware into a drawer. "You're not flopping down over here to sleep off your drunks."

I returned to the kitchen.

"Yes, of course you're right," she said sarcastically over her shoulder. "Hack Singletree's far too busy to waste his time with practical jokes. Unless, of course, he could squeeze in a little time between his morning at the stock exchange, his lunch with clients, and his afternoon board meeting."

She had me there. From what I'd gathered from rumor, Hack always seemed to have as much time as he wanted to do whatever he wanted. It was common knowledge that the principal didn't show up at the school for days at a time. "No," I said, "he wouldn't do that to me. Why should he?"

"Be-cause you are a *Yan*-kee," she said, exaggerating her elocution. "It's open season on Yankees in Grady County. You don't belong here, and you don't want to be here. Everybody knows that. You're here because you took a wrong turn and your car broke down. You're so desperate to leave, you fell for that reconstructive surgery crap from that phoney quack Barker. You're just like all those other academic assholes who use the 'pursuit of truth' as a rationalization for deserting the sick and needy."

"Shelly . . . ."

"You'll hang around until somebody pisses up your rope and blinds you with another line of bullshit that you can charge out to Hollywood and customize tits and bob noses in the name of science."

"I came back," I reminded her, "before bobbing a single tit."

"It didn't work out and you came back to your holding pattern, where you can sit around thumbing through the classified ads of the *New England Journal of Medicine* with eyes too glazed to read the fine print until another three-piece-suit yanks your chain. When you finally do flash ass on out of here, you'll brag at those Washington cocktail parties about being a missionary of the backwoods South." She drew in a long breath, the air hissing through her clenched teeth. "But let me ask you this," she said. "When you found the footprints, did you follow them? Did you try to track the monster to its lair, or did you just discover the tracks, then turn around and leave?"

"No," I admitted, "we didn't follow them. It was late; I knew I was coming here for supper. Listen, we don't have to do this. I'm just late. I'm sorry I'm just a little late. I'm sorry your souffle fell, but it's not like I betrayed you with another woman or gambled away the mortgage money."

"You don't *have* a mortgage," she reminded me. This train was headed down a familiar track, the question of commitment and mortgage. The last time I asked Shelly to marry me, she had answered, "I don't marry renters." Commissioner Worthy and his wife Ida had offered to sell me my quarters, the farmhouse on Lake Loonie, for almost no down payment and about the same small payments I was making to rent it, but I'd declined. The Worthys wanted another doctor in the county desperately enough to take a substantial real estate loss, and Shelly figured anybody sincere about putting down roots would have some earth, some land, to put them in. A Southerner's ties to the soil, I'd guessed, was at the bottom of Shelly making such an issue about the status of the whereabouts I infrequently rested my weary head.

"Shelly," I'd argued, "I know of hundreds, maybe thousands of people who live productive lives and produce generations of children on property they don't actually own."

"So do I," she had countered. "They are called squatters and sharecroppers." It did little good to remind her that she herself had plans to leave Grady for Vanderbilt Law School, pending finances. Of course, Vanderbilt was four-hundred miles away. Presumably, law school didn't pronounce the doom on our love affair and lives together since Shelly planned to practice in Grady or, if she had to, Flint. Being married to a lawyer was going to take some getting used to. Doctors and lawyers made dubious bedfellows, and Shelly would have been even more infuriated to know that Hack and I had discussed her at length on the mossy creek bank, passing a flask and waxing philosophically on many subjects. Bullshitting, Hack called it. Perhaps because of my isolation from male friendship, I'd dropped my usual urban and professional aloofness and warmed up to the bucolic schoolteacher, tolerating his views concerning my life. "Miss Shelly's nesting," he said. "That's what ladies do when they get sexually mature. And this thing about law school," he continued, "is probably just something to *fall back* on." It seemed to me more logical to *fall back* on a vocation that required less academic preparation, say ambulance driving. "Well, that just goes to show you got a lot to learn about women in general and about Miss Shelly in particular." We didn't broach the subject of Beulah Parker, whose dangerous eyes beguiled without revealing character. How different from Shelly's eyes, whose power to attract lay in bright flashes of anger, excitement, joy, and love. Beulah, I sensed, was a taboo subject.

"Well, I guess I've worn out my welcome here," I said to Shelly's back and the sink. "I've got a long day at the hospital tomorrow, so I'd better be going." I shifted from one foot to the other, hoping that she would turn slowly, her eyes overbrimming with remorseful tears, reaching to embrace me with sudsy forearms and covering my waiting mouth with hotly passionate kisses. Ha! She didn't. She didn't even offer to drive me home in the ambulance, but Clarice followed me to the mailbox, the loose skin of her mournful face pulling half moons into the bottoms of her eyeballs, commiserating my departure with a half-hearted AWROOOP that broke off into a yawn. Then she padded loosely back to the kitchen door as I set out on the two mile hike to Loonie Lake, Hack's unadulterated moonshine gnawing away at the lining of my stomach.

Walking home in the cool spring air, I realized that I was going to have to face the fact that my relationship with Shelly had become more volatile since that call from Hollywood and my interview in L.A. She knew my shortcomings, knew that I lacked the courage, confidence, and conviction to make the transition from the university to the *sticks*. She accepted as inevitable our eventual separation, realizing my need to return to the relative safety of an important academic medical institution. She accused me of having the messianic syndrome, the epidemic of altruism among idealistic young medical school students who believed they were destined to save the world. Indeed it was easier to play God in a university setting where I could climb the pedestal than it was here among the unwashed and howling masses who needed and deserved a good doctor.

Shelly thought I needed to grow up, and that was that. She saw my immaturity, my inadequate sense of mission and self, as the bugbear that threatened our future together. She didn't think anybody could have a sense of *self* without a sense of *place*. Both she and Hack viewed intelligence in terms of successful adaptation to environment, a sort of kick-ass Darwinism that made me a man without a country, who would be just as easily lured by the next scam as I was the last.

Of course, it would infuriate Shelly to be told that she thought like Hack on any subject. She wanted me to "grow up," to find my proper place in the Grady community. She didn't see my drinking moonshine with idle loafers and searching for swamp monsters as an auspicious sign. I ambled along in the moonlight, tired, hungry, and bummed out, sinking from the euphoria of strong drink.

Chapter Nine
(12 February 1983 Lake Loonie)

Appropriately enough, the telephone call from Hollywood, California--the one that should have alerted Shelly that maybe I wasn't the dog worth betting on to go the distance--had interrupted our lovemaking on the first Saturday after we had expressed and consummated our undying affection for one another.

There was an oak fire in the bedroom fireplace, and the wind moaned and rattled my old farmhouse. We were thrilled by the rare, cold weather and the excuse to have a fire. "Uh, hello," I answered. Shelly, her breasts heaving, rolled her eyes and placed the back of her hand on her forehead.

"Otis Stone? This is Dr. Steve Barker. How are you?"

Dr. Steve Barker was a senior resident during my internship at Jackson Memorial in Miami. Almost always moonlighting, almost never teaching, Barker was remarkable for ostentatious affluence, even in those days--his BMW, his Rollex, and his five-hundred-dollar suits. What on Earth did he want with me? "Nice to hear from you, Dr. Barker. How'd you find me?" I asked. This was a telephone call from an *actual medical doctor* in the *real* world.

"I've made it a point to keep up with you, Dr. Stone. Did I ever tell you you have a great set of hands?"

"Uh, no." Shelly bit me just above the kneecap, and I cleared my throat.

"Well, you do, and I'm also serious when I say, of all the interns I've ever taught, you're the brightest by far. You graduated number two at Stanford, didn't you? See, I remember."

"What can I do for you, Dr. Barker?" Even though I had regarded Steve Barker as an asshole, I couldn't help puffing up a little under his flattery. I couldn't make myself call him by his first name either.

"Well, essentially, I was just tracking you down, but I do have a proposition for you. As soon as I heard we had an opening, you were the first name that popped into my mind."

"Where are you calling from?"

"I'm out in Hollywood, California. I've got an interesting situation out here now," said Dr. Barker, "which is why I called you. Listen Stone, you need to have a look at our operation. I can offer you a fellowship and, listen to this, we'll match whatever you're making at, uh, Trafford Memorial. You'll be doing big things here, reconstructive surgery and research on the cutting edge. We're developing a major oncology/research center coupled with a reconstructive plastic surgery center. We expect to rival Sloan Kettering or M.D. Anderson. We want to be the Mayo of the West. After reconstruction, our mastectomy patients are going to look better than they did before they contracted cancer. So will our melanoma and head and neck cancer patients. How does that sound to you?" Suddenly my connection went bad. It sounded like Barker was stirring Irish stew with the receiver.

"Dr. Barker? Dr. Barker, are you still there?"

"And you'll love L.A. Lots of tinsel, lots of fringe."

"Fringe?"

"Sure, by the way what happened to your little blond nurse in Miami? Is she still with you?"

"She stayed."

"With you? Or in Miami?"

"There."

"Too bad, but there are plenty of girls out here. As a matter of fact there's a starlet standing here leaning against me with an unbelievably voluptuous conjunction of mammary glands, and guess who engineered those resplendent breasts?"

I couldn't believe I was having this conversation. *Conjunction*? *Mammary glands*? But I guessed I was, evidenced by the fact that I was calling Steve Barker "Doctor," a residual of the god-to-mortal supremacy the senior resident has over the intern. We imbued our superiors with power we hoped to assume somewhere down the line. What was he doing in California?

"YOU did?" I said. "YOU engineered the resplendent breasts?"

Shelly put her ear to the back of the receiver, the top of her head touching mine.

"My hospital did, but say hello to Miss Ruby Knight."

"Hello, Otis," said a husky female voice. "Doctor Barker says you've got a nice pair of hands."

Shelly twisted the receiver and flattened her warm ear against my jaw. I pushed her away. "Uh, thank you, Ruby."

"Who's that?" hissed Shelly, crawling back on her hands and knees and arching her back.

"Would you put Dr. Barker back on the phone, Ruby?" I requested, holding up an index finger to Shelly, then a palm.

Gurgling sounds assaulted my ear from long distance, and I began to think that Dr. Barker was abusing some substance, maybe Ruby, even as we spoke. He came back on, laughing and coughing.

"Look, get somebody to cover for you and come out for a few days. I'm sending you a round trip ticket to L.A. Here, write this down and get in touch as soon as you arrange for four or five days as our guest, all expenses paid, of course."

"Guess what, Shelly," I said after I hung up.

"Somebody massaged your ego and suckered you out to L.A.?"

"Don't be negative, Shelly. This could be *it*. This could be a shot at the big time, the cutting edge of oncological research, tah-dah, the Nobel Prize." I danced naked around the room, trying to pull her with me. "You'll love California. L.A. is rated very high in the Rand McNally Quality of Life index. California has everything, mountains, seashore, shopping malls, streetlights, indoor plumbing . . . ."

"Crime, smog, traffic . . . but NOT me," she said soberly. "I'll keep my flat feet on steady ground that doesn't quake or slide. Nearly everybody in Grady County has indoor plumbing, and I bet your doctor friend wears enough gold chains around his neck to pull a pulpwood truck out of a ditch."

I laughed.

Shelly got serious. "You have to go, don't you?" she said. "I guess I want you to."

"I have to check it out," I admitted. "It would haunt me if I didn't. It's a private hospital getting research dollars from the National Cancer Institute and turning big profits they can pump into high tech research. It's a chance for a prestigious job at a major academic center."

Shelly smiled, a beautiful, wise woman. "I guess I can understand that. Who'll take care of your patients?"

My patients. Somehow I hadn't thought of myself yet as a doctor with actual patients that needed me. I guess I still thought of myself as temporary, filling in for somebody else.

"You, Flowers, and Margaret Holt." Dr. Hogue was supposed to be convalescing from his January 31 heart attack, but he could not break his habit of being Grady's only doctor. He still treated me like a medical technician, which was less condescending than his regard for Lee Bob Parker and Sherman Flowers, upon whose mention he just sadly shook his head, but I wasn't a finished product in his estimation, not by a long shot. "Anything real serious, Flowers can confer with Dr. Hogue and refer to Putnam Memorial, and you can drive them over." Sherman Flowers was the creepy emergency room M.D. Dr. Hogue and I had imported from New Orleans without looking too closely at his credentials. Shelly and I were both sure he was using his narcotics key to supply himself with Dilaudid, and we suspected him of writing prescriptions out to a cadaverous looking belladonna who drove her '75 T-Bird regularly into the ER parking lot.

"Flowers will refer anything serious to Harland Hooks," Shelly said. Hooks was the mortician who, it was quipped without much levity, buried Flowers' mistakes.

To her credit, possessiveness wasn't in Shelly's nature. She couldn't help getting excited over my imagined good fortune, even if it meant the end of our affair, and she shared my contagious good spirits. When the airplane ticket arrived, she helped me pack and drove me to Flint Airport, which connected me north to Atlanta and on to Tinseltown, U.S.A. "Watch out for Ruby!" Shelly called as I boarded the air shuttle to Atlanta.

I kept expecting the good citizens of Grady, under the leadership of Ida Worthy, to try to abort my departure. I waited for Sheriff Bootman to arrive at the airport with some phony writ, warrant, or summons to stay my departure. In the past Grady residents had shown considerable resourcefulness to prevent my leaving. They'd refused to extend credit, they'd created phoney debts, denied being able to fix my car, served me fried chicken dinners, and presented me a lifetime membership in the trap and skeet club. They'd done everything short of actually incarcerating me in the county jail. But now they figured I'd have to come back for Shelly, and they could jail me then. Maybe they thought I'd spent enough time in the county to feel that I belonged there. Hack summed it up a year later, "Keep a stole chicken long enough, she'll roost with the thief."

As it happened, Hollywood's bright lights did not lure me away from Grady. In the first place, I longed for Shelly like an adolescent, calling her at home and work under the guise of professional concern for my patients--whom I surprised myself by worrying over every moment I wasn't longing for Shelly. In the second place, Dr. Barker turned out to be a phoney, his operation--a multi-million dollar scam. When I returned from L.A. two days earlier than planned, disillusioned, disappointed, and despondent, Shelly was there, dressed in maroon trousers and white shirt, to greet me and share my professional grief.

My return flight barked its tires on the runway and taxied in. Shelly stood at the terminal, holding a single red rose which clashed with her polyester trousers. Even uniformed like a bellhop, she was the prettiest thing I'd ever seen. I swore I'd make her come with me next time, no matter what I had to promise. We both ran, meeting halfway between the airplane and the terminal. She threw her arms around me, kissing me wantonly and scratching my neck with a thorn. "Ouch!"

"Couldn't you tell it was too good to be true, Stone?" she said as she drove me home. I could tell she was happy. She drove like a maniac, sucking up white lines. A death wish. The drab winter landscape was patched with lush green fields of winter rye.

"I guess this is when girl tells boy 'I told you so,'" I said.

"Well, I told you so," she smiled. The ambulance leaned away from a wide curve.

"That, you did."

"When did you find out?"

40

"It started smelling fishy pretty quick. Barker picked me up in a BMW sedan. He was wearing dark glasses and was attached at the hip to a red-headed model with legs that started at her earrings. She was supposed to take me anywhere I wanted to go if I couldn't get Barker. It wasn't Ruby."

Shelly raised her eyebrows.

"Then at the hospital there were lots of five-pound glass ashtrays. Three quarters of the doctors were Asian Indians named Patel trying to get board certified. Barker was cherry-picking talent for cheap labor to do scut work."

"Which is?" Shelly was watching the road, a good thing since we were traveling faster than 85 mph on the flat two-lane between Flint and Grady. I was watching the speedometer.

"Somebody to do histories and physical exams and to follow up on medical problems. They do some token mastectomies and head and neck reconstructions, just enough to keep their certification and qualify for National Cancer Institute bucks. They use cancer patients for guinea pigs to develop technology for cosmetics. For every cancer patient there are 10 cosmetics, and there's plenty of opportunity for expansion in Tinsel and where physical perfection is the norm and Mother Nature's products are believed to be flawed from birth. Hollywood is the plastic surgery capital of the world."

"I'll bet it wasn't all those flawless bodies that scourged you home."

"Nope, I finally insisted on reviewing the annual report, which revealed the secrets of those philanthropic hearts. Last year two million went to research. The head honcho's salary was 2.5 million. Even rock stars shouldn't make that kind of money."

"Not even the Rolling Stones?"

"Well, maybe the Rolling Stones."

"What were they going to pay you?" When we passed the Grady County line, Shelly slowed down. She liked speed, but she had sacrificed her excuse now that the ambulance was back in the county.

"Forty thousand."

"Humm."

"They found out what I was making when they found out where I was. That or they called around. They went down an alumni roster from Jackson Memorial Hospital in Miami. They were pyramiding ten doctors into two plastic surgeon slots, getting their scut work done. But it was a dream that finally sent me packing. The money would have been O.K. if the hospital had been what Barker said it was. I thought I was going to get to the academic big time. They bring in ten times more fellows than they can certify at the end of eight years. For the first two years the internists study oncology with the promise of moving up to plastic surgery for another six years. It's a pyramid scam. They can certify in general surgery slots, but their program isn't accredited for oncology or plastic surgery, so the only way you can get board certified in surgery is by staying for eight years and beating out the other ten guys. The odds are ten to one of getting zilch accreditation."

"You mean you could waste eight years."

"Well, you'd probably see the light and drop out before then."

"Which is what you did. But I want to hear about your dream. What are one's visions when one is surrounded by flawless bodies and cocaine?"

"I dreamed about Carl Hogue."

"I don't believe it." She turned and squinted. "You were totally immersed in starlets, and you dreamed about Dr. Hogue. By the way, he came back to work."

"You're kidding. Now there's one man out to kill himself. He should be in bed another six weeks. Anyway, Dr. Hogue comes to me like the Spirit of Christmas Past, with floating hair, but he's in Hollywood. Like he's worked 35 years at Barker's hospital instead of spending his life as Grady's only real doctor. I hear his voice, distant and reedy, as from the grave saying: 'I am personally responsible for ten thousand impeccable tits, eight thousand face lifts, two thousand tummy tucks, and a quarter mile of trimmed noses.'"

"Are you sure he said 'tits'? 'Tits' doesn't sound like Dr. Hogue."

"I'm positive. It shocked me too."

"Are you sure he said 'impeccable'"?

"I *think* he said 'impeccable,' but that wasn't all. There was this parade of flabby body parts, like Salvador Dali's watches--breasts, nose tips, faces. But that wasn't the worst part. The worst part was an Asian Indian named Patel stirring an enormous vat of oil with a canoe paddle. He winks and says it's residue from the liposuctions."

"Yuck, how do you know he was named Patel?"

"All the Indian doctors were named Patel. It's a caste name, but this one has a blue plastic name tag and dark circles around his eyes. He says he's saving the fat for waterbeds. I think that part of the dream came from a surreal medical supply salesman I met at a party. He had a special king-size frame full of silicone implants--factory rejects, I guess."

"Wow," said Shelly, "I wonder what that was like."

"He said it was cold at first until a few starlets dived in and squirmed around. Then the silicon warmed up and it was like returning to the womb or getting swallowed by a whale--they're all Freudians out there. The secret is getting somebody to go in ahead of you."

"Like with everything else." She cocked her head.

"He's still trying to figure a way to warm it up first, maybe with an electric blanket."

"Well, I'm proud of you."

"For not inviting myself into the rep's star-studded bed?"

"That and for coming home and turning your back on all that fame and fortune, for not staying out there to liposuck and live off the fat of the land, so to speak."

"Well, when the airplane was circling for a landing a few minutes ago, I did have the distinct feeling of coming down to earth."

"I missed you, and I'm glad you're home."

"Me too," I said, taking her hand, then putting it quickly back on the steering wheel. "You were right about the gold chains too. Barker had a silk shirt unbuttoned at the neck with a gold Krugerrand. Everybody was into gold chains, coke, chrome furniture, and Pre-Columbian art."

"Well, we still have a few sick human beings in Grady for you to work on, Doctor. I think we can find something here for you to do for people who are anatomically similar to Californians. I don't think I would have fit into L.A. society."

I tousled her hair. "Sure you would. I'd buy you a mini skirt, add a gold coke spoon to your charm bracelet, and you'd be fine. Maybe some false eyelashes." I suddenly realized that my disappointment had dissipated. And even against the pewter February sky, my spirits began to soar. Shelly had that effect on me.

Chapter Ten

W hen Dr. Hogue died, I became the captain of a sinking ship. His death shouldn't have come as a surprise. His bouts of angina had increased in frequency since his January 31st heart attack. I'd tried to sit him down and discuss his electrocardiogram with him, but he'd dismissed the particulars of his own condition--knowing well what the symptoms indicated--as though his lifetime dedication to the practice of medicine had immunized him against disease. He began seeing patients against my advice, and he had a fatal heart attack while pumping X-lax out of Billy Oaks' stomach. The old family practitioner hadn't trusted me even with the stomach pump. Ironically, I had to finish up the Oaks kid with Dr. Hogue slumped in his chair, monitoring me with astonished, sightless eyes, one nearly twice the size of the other. "What's wrong with Dr. Hogue?" Billy Oaks asked when I removed the tubes. Hogue was already cold. I wondered how Billy had managed to remain still with a tube down his throat for so long, but then assumed Dr. Hogue's stern supervisory stare accounted for Billy's cooperative demeanor.

"He's tired," I said. "He worked too long and too hard and he's tired."

I ushered Billy to his mother and returned to a dead family practitioner. "I could have left Grady," I told him. "With you still alive, I could have gone. But now I'm stuck. There's nobody here but me."

Hogue looked as though he wanted to answer but couldn't quite frame the words. His expression was like the one on the old cardboard effigy of Uncle Sam in front of the post office, the one that pointed a finger and tracked you with accusatory, owlish eyes saying, "Uncle Sam needs you." I felt like the reluctant prince after the king has died and left him a kingdom nobody knows how to run. Before Hogue's death I could have moved on, maybe found a fellowship and managed to save face. But not now. There was no way. Not unless I found a family practitioner to replace Hogue. I was, as Hack would put it, between a rock and a hard place. I wasn't the doctor they needed, but I was the only one they had. I'd be an internist following in the footsteps of a family physician who was licensed to do everything. I could recognize symptoms, diagnose illness, and refer patients to specialists, but I was also bound by ethical restrictions against practicing the kind of comprehensive medicine Grady needed. I wasn't licensed to do *any*thing. I couldn't enter areas where I wasn't board certified. I lacked the credentials and experience for the kind of nuts-and-bolts medicine needed in an underserved area. My training was hopelessly inadequate.

"Who you talkin' to?" demanded Margaret Holt, barging through the door. "What ail Dr. Hogue?" Then instantly she saw and knew. She stood there solid and truculent until her bottom lip began to tremble. I walked over to her and wrapped my arms around her as far as they would reach. I held her a long time. Her great body shuddered as she sobbed, absorbing her grief. Dr. Hogue was more than just an old friend and mentor to Margaret Holt, he was the institution of medicine--past, present, and future. He was the force that held the hospital together, the reason for Margaret's having a job as head nurse, her profession.

Thus Hogue's death opened the floodgates of professional frustration and despair. I wasn't prepared to handle most emergencies or treat the majority of patients who came to me for help. I wasn't licensed to set broken bones, perform appendectomies, remove gall bladders, or treat children, but my inability to deliver babies weighed on me the heaviest. We called ourselves miracle workers. What was a country doctor worth, even a reluctant country doctor, who couldn't deliver a baby?

Carl Hogue had delivered some five thousand babies in a county whose present population was only fifteen thousand souls. He had set three thousand bones, taken out five hundred gall bladders. He would have consoled four thousand families. How many people's lives had he overseen during his thirty-odd years of family practice? From the cradle to the grave, from womb to tomb, he played an essential role in the lives of thousands of people.

I knew I was destined to feel a great deal of inadequacy after his death, when my self-esteem suffered an all time low and my training had little application to Grady's needs. I believe I would have sneaked out of town if I'd had a car. Nurse Holt's tears had soaked my lab coat from nape to shoulder.

Chapter Eleven

C'mon back!" Four mobile homes, repossessions on loan from the Chairman of the Grady County Commission Bill Worthy, were being positioned on a lot belonging to the City of Grady. "Moan back!" Commissioner Worthy yelled to the bucktoothed man on a green tractor, which spurted a plume of black smoke.

A yellow school bus with bars on the windows showed up with a crew of prisoners from the county jail. Sheriff Bootman, foreseeing the need for skilled labor, raided a cockfight and was able to arrest a half dozen skilled construction workers, including the foreman, on drunkenness in a public place, disorderly conduct, and gambling charges. Bootman's prisoners grumbled that they didn't see how Felix Mayberry's barn came to be called a public place. He dried them out in jail and had Judge Savage sentence them to community service "for a term not to exceed the completion of the Grady Medical Arts complex."

Men in prison jump suits milled around laughing and cutting up with a guard, who had a cheek full of chewing tobacco and a shotgun over his shoulder. It was a clear March day with white windswept clouds against a high blue sky. The prisoners couldn't hold a grudge, even for conscription, on such a day. The Commissioner and his civic-minded wife, Miss Ida Worthy, were both on the premises. The commissioner stood erect, supervising with hands in his pockets and a cigar in his mouth. Miss Ida was wearing Liberty overalls and mule hide gloves, a staple gun in one hand and a hammer in the other. I was sure that no two citizens in the history of medicine were more intent on having a doctor in their county.

"This is essentially a chain gang," I protested. "It's illegal."

"Them boys ain't wearing no chains is the difference between this and a chain gang," said Miss Ida, who had marched over to ask what colors I wanted for the waiting room interior. "And they'd heap rather be out here in the sunshine than sitting in jail collecting mildew, which reminds me . . . I got you a surprise."

"Maybe I don't want to know about it."

"Come over here, Rooster Bootman!" she called to the sheriff.

After Dr. Hogue's death I had tried to buy his office. I couldn't get a clear title because the collateral was tied up in a local trust, with Karl Wright as beneficiary. The trust had come as a surprise to Buster and Mrs. Hogue too. The good doctor had borrowed against his practice to keep medicine in Grady solvent. Now, except for a modest insurance settlement, he had passed that legacy of sacrifice on to his family.

I had thought at first that Karl Wright would be only too glad to sell me Dr. Hogue's office at a reasonable price, but I found out very quickly through

Wright's attorney Morton Willetts that Doctors Holding and Managing Company in Atlanta owned the accounts receivable and corporate assets. It seemed that somebody had made a deliberate effort to prevent another doctor from using the building for an office, which I found out later was exactly what Willetts and Wright had in mind. I didn't discover until after New Years, nine months later, that Wright wanted to buy Trafford and convert it to an out-patient surgery center for Southern Vision. To do that it was in his best interests to keep any new doctors out of Grady. New doctors would mean an increased hospital census and improved financial status, and Wright wanted to put Trafford on its financial knees and pick it up at a bargain basement price. The push-pin flag in his library map was no accident after all. He was a smart and sleazy corporate raider. His tactics had worked at other rural southwest Georgia hospitals, but he had underestimated Grady County's determination to have health care for its citizens.

The sheriff came over to me and Miss Ida, removing his hat.

"Thomas Freelander over yonder's from Corrections," he said. "He's doing life for murder, but the judge got him released in your custody while he's laying your masonry, but you got to go down and sign some papers. He's a expert mason. That's his grand-youngun helping him. He wants to teach him the trade."

"Wait a minute, Sheriff," I said. "I can't be responsible for a murderer." Freelander had already crossed off a large area with stakes and string.

"Thomas ain't no murderer," Bootman said defensively. "He killed somebody is all."

"I can't be responsible for a killer either, and the distinction eludes me." I had to admit the old man with his grandson didn't look much like a coldblooded killer, knocking old mortar joints from used bricks with his trowel and stacking the bricks in a neat pile. Miss Ida returned to work while Bootman filled me in on my recognizant brick layer.

Thomas Freelander had been convicted of what law enforcement officers called a misdemeanor murder. In the typical misdemeanor murder, the killer calls the police to report the crime. When they arrive he says, "Here's the body. Here's the knife. I'm the one done it. Let me get my coat and lock up the house."

"It was a crime of passion," explained Bootman. "Most of us got one murder in us. Thomas over there's done got his out of his system, so he's safer to walk the streets than you and me, who ain't had our murder yet. There was likely only one man in Georgia able to make Thomas mad enough to kill, and that man ain't around no more as a temptation."

I'd heard that Southern cops view blacks killing blacks less seriously than other murder. I couldn't help asking, "Did Thomas kill another black man or a white?"

"He killed his son-in-law, who was sorry as gully dirt. He was bad to drink and beat up Bonita, Thomas' daughter. Thomas goes to him, says 'Listen here Monroe, you married my girl, but you ain't got nothing in her. I'm the one raised her up, put braces on her teeth, and bought her food and clothes. If she don't please you, bring her on back to my house and we'll call it even. But you ever lay another hand on her, I'm gone put you in the ground.' Six months later Bonita goes to the hospital, and the next day Thomas comes down to my office and hands me his claw hammer."

"Claw hammer?"

"The murder weapon. Thomas rattles Monroe's screen door, and when Monroe opens it, Thomas punches a hole the size of a plum in the middle of his forehead."

"Monroe's flopping like a mud cat on his front porch when my deputy, Jim Marshall, gets there. Monroe is dead before he falls, but he keeps on flopping. The driver from Stokes has to strap him on the stretcher to keep him from hopping off." Bootman smiled. "Jim finds Thomas walking down the road with the hammer in his hand. He pulls up beside him and asks him where he's going, and Thomas says he's going to see me. The deputy asks him does he want a ride, and Thomas says no thank you. The deputy radios me and asks what to do. 'Did he say he was coming in?' I says. 'That's what he says,' goes Jim Marshall. 'Well, let him come head on then,' I says. Says, 'You follow him, but don't crowd him. Don't get so close it looks like you herding him down here.'"

"By the time Thomas gets to town, the streets are lined with folks, same as for a parade. Thomas, walking tall and looking straight ahead, climbs the courthouse steps, comes in my office and hands me the claw hammer across my desk. He sits in a straightback chair while I read him his rights. Then he asks can he use my bathroom to clean up where Monroe's blood has done spattered his glasses. There ain't nothing else for the jury to do but convict him of premeditated murder, since Thomas had been meditating on murdering that sum-bitch since the first time he laid a hand on Bonita. Turns out Monroe did have something in Bonita, though. That boy yonder, Monroe's son, was in her belly when Thomas tapped the daddy into the next life."

I watched Freelander half a brick with a sharp chop from the edge of his trowel. He handed the trowel and another brick to his teenage grandson, who tried to half the brick and couldn't. Freelander lifted a brick hammer from the loop in his overalls and showed the grandson how to half a brick with the blade face of the hammer.

"Anyway," Rooster continued, "wait till you see what he's planning to make this place into. I seen the drawings he made. It'll look like the Tasha's Mall."

"What?"

"It'll look real good."

Rooster led me over to Thomas Freelander, who with obvious pride introduced me to his grandson. Freelander was a tall, thin man with a strong handshake and a bullet shaped head covered with white stubble. He held a brick bat in one hand and was adding water to the cement mortar his grandson was mixing in a wheelbarrow with a hoe.

The plans for Thomas' masonry work were drawn in painstaking detail in pencil on a three-foot section of butcher paper. They included a four-foot wall around the entire property, a fresh air gazebo for an outdoor waiting area, and a patio. Freelander had drawn in brick skirting and steps for the trailers, walkways, a brick mailbox and fountain. "This will take months," I observed. "Where will he get the bricks?"

"Ida Worthy will get him ever brick in Grady he needs. Those bricks there come out the bomb shelter they built in 1957 behind the courthouse. Everbody thought the Russians was going to drop atomic bombs on Grady, Georgia. You too young to remember air raid drills when a siren would go off and the teachers made the school kids get up under their desks. Like that desk was gone save them kids from a atomic blast," Rooster grinned. "It ain't no wonder everbody forty years old is crazy as a squirrel. Speaking of which, yonder comes Hack Singletree. Now there's a man got one murder left in him, maybe two."

Hack's green truck tilted to the driver's side on worn out shocks. It rattled to a stop. Hack swung out and lifted a cardboard box from the bed. "I got your filing system," he announced.

In Hack's box were three wooden blocks with a ten-penny nail hammered through each. They were painted white and stenciled in red letters: IN, OUT, and MISCELLANEOUS. "Keep it simple," Hack advised. "If the unforseen occurs, I'll hunt you up another block."

"He ain't teasing," Rooster Bootman said. "That's the way he runs the junior high. When his IN spike gets more than his OUT, he shoots stickbirds and fights chickens with the IN till the spikes balance out."

"After you finish up here," Hack asked Thomas Freelander, "how'd you like a job teaching at the junior high? You look like a man who knows a weep-hole from a tinker's dam."

A dark Lincoln Town Car pulled up to the curb. The driver tapped the horn and zipped down the electric window on the passenger side. Commissioner Bill Worthy walked over and leaned into the window without removing his cigar as Hack leaned over to pick up one of Thomas Freelander's brick bats, winding up as if to throw. The window zipped shut, almost catching the commissioner's head, and the Lincoln jerked away from the curb. "Karl Wright," grinned Hack. "A pluperfect son-of-a-bitch."

Chapter Twelve
(May 1983)

So I was a country doctor unable to deliver babies. Yet, as Shelly sagely observed, babies continued being born, assisted by midwives or simply arriving while husbands shifted weight from one foot to the other, twisting their hats. Some mothers at term, unable to afford hospital obstetrics, waited until the penultimate moment and dashed to the emergency room to be delivered by Margaret Holt, assisted by Shelly or Buster, who had matured even in the few short weeks since his father's death. It seemed more than a little ironic that nurses and EMT's were given more latitude than I, an internist, was allowed.

Sometimes the miracle of life asserted itself urgently, as it did later that March when Shelly answered a *boondocks* call alone. She pulled into the swept-dirt yard of a tenant house at the end of an unpaved road, where barefoot adults and children waved her in. The mother, a child herself at fourteen, was attended by her grandmother. "They coming," the grandmother said, "and I believes they's more than one." Shelly secured the expectant mother on the stretcher in the back of the ambulance and set out for the hospital whirling red dust, but when she heard the young mother scream above the siren, Shelly slammed on brakes by a wet-weather pond, delivered two squalling infants and returned, at the mother's insistence, to the tenant house, where family and friends still moiling in the yard raised their hands, singing in celebration.

I found Shelly in the emergency room parking lot washing out the ambulance with a hose. Pink water dripped out the back door. Shelly's eyes were glazed. "You should have heard those peepers," she said, staring past me.

"What?"

"The peepers, the little frogs in the lilypond. The whole morning buzzed. The air was electric with them. I felt so . . . alive."

"I've never delivered twins," I said.

"Don't pout," she said. "There's nothing to it. It's just like receiving a snap from center except your dominant hand is down." She positioned her hands like a quarterback's. "Hup, two, three, push!"

"I'll have to remember that."

"Otis?"

"What?"

"Let's ride back out to the boonies so you can listen to the peepers."

"I'm on call."

"Of course you're on call. You're always on call. Who else is there now that Hogue's dead."

"There's Flowers?"

"Bring your beeper. Anyway, we'll go in the ambulance. It's got a radio."

"I know you," I said. "You just want to visit your 'duo.' You want to gloat."

"I might swing by there, yes." Her expression was powerful and serene. "Let's go," she said.

We entered the gray tenant house with the calico brick chimney. Rusty nails creaked as we climbed the plank steps and crossed a threshold worn by generations of bare feet. As we entered to visit Shellene and Shellyanne, namesakes of their intrepid deliverer, other household members went outside so we could privately visit the young mother Shasta, who breast fed the twins in the partial darkness of the single room. The room smelled sweet and rich with life. Shelly lifted Shellene as I spoke with Shasta, routinely asking postpartum platitudes.

"How are you feeling, Shasta?"

"Glad," she said, beaming.

"Glad?"

"Glad I got my babies. Glad I got Shellene and Shellyann."

"Well, what beside that?"

"Nothin' 'sides that," she smiled. "What else I 'spose to feel?"

"Well, I thought you might feel a little, uh, sore."

Shasta bubbled with laughter, loud adolescent giggles. "I do be some sore," she agreed watching Shelly lift a baby, holding the infant's head against the nape of her neck.

This black kid was laughing at me, and Shelly was too. I couldn't understand what they found so funny.

My place, indeed my generic male presence in that room, seemed superfluous. I was embarrassed about being there, frustrated by their unwillingness in their pure feminine happiness to acknowledge me or take me seriously.

"Well, that's normal," I added professionally.

Again Shasta giggled, joined by Shelly.

Still ill at ease, I changed the cant of my question from the professional to the humane. "Where's the proud papa?"

"My daddy dead."

"No, the baby's. The father of your child. Your husband."

"He somewhere in his socks, if he got some. Shellene and Shellyann aine got no daddy," Shasta smiled, "but they got them a mamma. Granmamma too."

———————

"I can't believe you asked that child about her husband," Shelly remarked as we pulled off the red clay road by the wet weather pond. "You're something else!"

"What's wrong with that?" I was still piqued about being laughed at.

"Fourteen-year-old children don't have husbands."

"Well, somebody biologically fathered that baby. Her paramour then."

"Fourteen-year-old children don't have paramours either," she smiled, that private sparkle in her eyes, "but twenty-seven-year-old women do."

We rolled down the windows of the cab to hear Shelly's peepers, but now the pond was silent. The surface was covered with glossy green lilypads. The woods beyond were tinged with the green-gold of new growth and the red of winged maple seeds, but the frogs didn't make a peep. We entered the back of the ambulance where Shelly had a bottle of Champagne chilled in a Little Oscar cooler originally intended for delivering severed appendages to the hospital.

"What's the occasion?" I asked. She handed me a stemmed plastic glass and ricochetted the cork off the defibrillator. She poured the wine and reached behind to unhook her bra.

"I want to christen the ambulance's first birth," she said. "And we're alive. It's springtime, and we're alive, and in love, even."

"I've never had sex in an ambulance before," I said. I expected her to say "me neither," but she didn't.

"There's nothing to it so long as it's parked and the emergency brake is on."

"Aw shucks, Shelly," I said in my best cornpone accent, nuzzling her neck where Shellene's tiny head had rested. The sweet odor of newborn baby lingered there.

"I love it when you talk dirty," she said.

––––––––––

When we climbed back out through the double doors of the ambulance, there was plenty of racket around the wet-weather pond. The peepers were sounding off and the cicadas joined in. My beeper beeped and the horn, which was connected to the radio, sounded as the radio spit static. Margaret Holt was calling to alert us that the Wiggins twins had swallowed a snot agate and three cat-eyes, which Shelly explained were marbles. A cow, another marble the size of a persimmon, had entered one twin's alimentary system from the posterior portal. We returned to the hospital.

Chapter Thirteen

I knew something like this would happen if they didn't stop playing keepsies," the harried mother sighed. Mrs. Wiggins, in the vernacular of the region, looked like she'd been rode hard and put up muddy, and the reasons for her perpetual fatigue were sitting side-by-side like gargoyles in Red Camel overalls. Ronald and Donald Wiggins were at nine years old dead serious identical twins who wore adult expressions of irredeemable depravity and crows feet of grime around their eyes. They had never smiled except from pleasure derived from torturing cats or frying caterpillars with a magnifying glass. Anyone believing in the prelapsarian innocence of children hadn't met the Wiggins twins, who were born bad to the bone. "What's keepsies?" I asked Margaret Holt.

"You never played marbles?" she said, looking down her nose at me, the alien.

"Uh, uh."

Buster stepped forward. His transformation in the six short weeks since his father's death had astounded us all. Released from Carl Hogue's umbrage, he experienced a spurt of emotional growth and maturity. He'd renounced his unrealistic aspirations of becoming a neurosurgeon, opting instead to concentrate on his EMT homework at Flint Junior College, where his vocabulary, at least, had begun to flourish. Buster's textbooks had accumulated in the ER lounge along with Shelly's law books and my journals. Among them I'd noticed a Roget's Thesaurus and several guides to vocabulary including one entitled *Powerhouse of Language: Dynamic Diction for Men*. He had also started spending more time with his mother and stopped trying to screw everything with a pulse. He cut his golden tresses into a sensible low-maintenance haircut and discontinued his lovelorn glances at Shelly. "Well," he began, "marbles belonging to both players are contained by a circle drawn in the dirt. Each player attempts to dislodge his opponent's marbles from the circle with his shooter, which is a marble cradled in the index finger and projected with the thumb. Keepsies is a game after which the opponent's marbles are not returned."

"The captured marbles aren't eaten, are they?"

"No," said Buster. "In this case, Ronald won Donald's favorite snot-agate, and Donald proposed that he surrender three cat eyes in their stead. Ronald refused and they fought, the scuffle resulting in Ronald's ingestion of the cat eyes and the snot agate. Donald in retribution inserted Ronald's cow into his own rectal orifice."

"He stuck it in his rectum?"

"Exactly. He crammed it up his ass."

Mrs. Wiggins cringed.

"Don't worry, Mrs. Wiggins, anything small enough to go in is small enough to come out.

"Give Ronald a dose of mineral oil," I told Margaret Holt. "Donald, you come back here with me."

Ronald's marbles would make their labyrinthine way through the esophagus, the stomach, the duodenum, the small intestines, the colon, exiting Ronald's vent into the toilet bowl.

But the cow was a slightly different story. It rested like a rifle ball in the breach of Donald's rectum, just above the anal sphincter, where it could be easily reached, removable with the aid of small spoonbill forceps, if I couldn't coax Donald into passing it.

I had Donald remove his overalls and assume a position on his elbows and knees. I hoped that this position of presented buttocks and lowered head would apply outward pressure against the marble, facilitating its removal. Actually Donald looked like a dwarf worshiping Islam.

"Don't try nothing funny, Doc." he said.

"Shut up, Donald."

The most immediate and obvious observation I made was that Donald paid even less attention to personal hygiene than most nine-year-old boys. "You have feces on your rectum!" I informed him.

"What's that?"

"Shit. You have shit on your ass, Donald!"

"Well, what'd you expect, Doc, sugar?"

"Just hold still." I put on a pair of latex gloves and cleaned Donald up with a surgical sponge; then I spread his cheeks and peered into his anus. Nothing. I probed with my index finger.

"I don't like that!" Donald snapped, trying to look back at me.

"Good, you're not supposed to," I snapped back. I felt the hard, curved surface of the marble, but when I tried to reach behind it, it slid deeper into Donald. I removed my finger. "Push," I told him.

"What?"

"Push!"

"Push what?"

"Try to break wind."

"Fart?"

"Yes."

"Uhhhhh," said Donald.

The marble was moving. I could barely see it now deep inside Donald, shining dark green like a jewel in a god's eye. Each time Donald pushed, it moved closer. As he relaxed, the eye winked sardonically. Finally the cow crowned. "Hold it right there." I moved aside, resting one hand on the top of Donald's elevated buttocks and reaching with the other for a small pair of spoonbill forceps. Donald's face strained, his red cheeks puffed with air. "Hooooold it." I was about to lift the marble from its setting when I realized with sudden clarity that what was supposed to happen in the first place was happening now. Donald was launching his marble.

"Don't push!" I cried too late, stepping clear. The cow, fueled by an astonishing flatulence, was expelled, arching with a crack to the tile floor. It bounced three times, rattling and rolling out of sight.

"Boy!" exclaimed Donald, "Boy oh boy oh boy."

"Boy oh boy," I mimicked, picturing in my mind's eye the puffy clouds that would someday carry me away from all this to a university hospital in a real city. What the hell was I doing here in the first place? I was determined not to spend my career dodging anal projectiles from demented little yahoos with filthy rectums. I was through. Shelly could stay or she could go with me. But I was going to escalate my search for a replacement and get the hell out of Grady.

I ushered Donald into the ER waiting room, where Mrs. Wiggins was standing with uplifted eyes, like a tortured Christian martyr appealing to heaven for deliverance. Donald swaggered over to his brother, swollen with pride. "I fired that cow like a thirty-ought-six, didn't I Doc?"

"Indeed you did, Donald. Indeed you did."

———————

As I was leaving the hospital for the day, Lee Bob Parker, medical director of Lilies of the Field Nursing Home, sallied in wearing a yellow Izod shirt and golf shoes. When he walked he sounded like a goat chewing a windshield. Appropriately, Lee Bob skimmed extra income drawing blood from senior citizens, testing it in the hospital lab, and he made regular trips to Trafford under one guise or another to scout the wards for potential inmates. He had already heard about my marble extraction. He slapped me on the back and told me about a senile 89-year-old female patient at Lilies with a vaginal discharge. He had given her a pelvic examination and discovered a smiling set of dental plates nestled in her vagina. "Big mystery," said Parker, raising his eyebrows. "They weren't hers. I told the staff, 'Just look for a little old man gumming a smile.' Ha, ha, ha. The old timers are bad about that sort of thing."

Ha, ha, ha. No they're not, I thought. Old people in institutions that emphasize care instead of profits are *not* bad about that sort of thing. Jesus Christ, I hated that son-of-a-bitch. I was glad his wife slept around.

I went by Shelly's on the way home, and she surprised me with a shaker of

Martinis. I had forgotten drinks other than beer existed.

"How middle class is this?" she asked brightly, bringing in the pitcher and stemmed conical glasses.

"Just what the doctor ordered," I said. "It's been a singular day."

She poured, and I could feel the icy gin through my glass and see the delicious condensation.

"You are genuinely wonderful," I said. I really needed a drink, but just as I lifted the Martini to my lips, the red-eyed pimento-stuffed olive glared up at me from the bottom of the glass, seeming to wink as the gin rolled back and forth. I couldn't take the first sip. "But could I have a twist of lemon?"

The next day Margaret Holt greeted me with a small brown envelope, which she emptied into a sponge in the palm of her hand. "Mrs. Wiggins dropped them off for you." She laid them down.

On the sink four marbles rested on the gauze; three were bright blue and the other was cloudy with a milky swirl. I pointed to the milky marble."That would be the, uh . . . ."

"Snot agate!" Mrs. Holt snapped.

"What do I want with them?"

"Mrs. Wiggins say you want them sent to the lab."

"Why would I send marbles to the lab?"

"I don't know why you want them marbles sent to the lab. I'm just a nurse. Maybe you want to have them tested for a malignancy, Doctor, which won't surprise me none."

"You are the *head* nurse of this hospital, Mrs. Holt, and capable of discretion and discrimination. You don't send marbles, not even snot-agates, to the lab to have them tested for malignancy."

"Mrs. Wiggins say you told her to watch for them marbles. She do and she brings them here, and here they is. I don't know what you want with them marbles. And I don't care. I'm just a nurse. You can throw them away, study them, lag to the line, play keepsies, send them to the lab, or you can stuff them where Donald put his cow. But don't you never tell me nothing about discrimination because there's a heap of things you do around here don't make a bit sense to me." Mrs. Holt's fists were on her hips, her feet were planted firmly, and her bosom swelled.

It wasn't a good time to confront her, if there ever was a good time. I turned, heading for the doctors' lounge, but she wasn't finished.

"I'm head nurse of something," she shouted, "but it ain't no hospital. Some kind of referral agency is what this is. All I'm doing is shuffling papers and sending sick folks to Putnam Memorial!" Margaret Holt was a good woman and a fine nurse. She missed Carl Hogue acutely, and she hated seeing her hospital collapse around her. Perhaps her sauciness was misplaced loyalty for Dr. Hogue. I was sorry I'd snapped at her about the marbles, but in my paranoia I was positive she was impudently reminding me of my insignificance as a healer. Later I would learn that the bighearted and bellicose Margaret Holt was utterly incapable of subtlety. Margaret Holt was about as subtle as an iron mace. The next day I sent an apologetic bouquet of flowers to her station. The flowers didn't make her smile, but they reduced the swelling in her lower lip. Sooner or later, Margaret Holt and I were going to have to bury the hatchet.

Chapter Fourteen

Hack Singletree was an ink addict, without being erudite. He was as irresistibly drawn to the label on the catsup bottle at the cafe as the steamiest best-selling novel. He didn't love literature or discriminate the contents of what he read. What was before him he devoured, moving his lips, sometimes mumbling aloud, following the lines with a blunt finger. He didn't enjoy, as most avid readers do, discussing subject matter. He found everything irresistible, nothing remarkable, and his disease was complicated by raging insomnia. He'd read the telephone book if there was no other material nearby. He'd read the Holy Bible numerous times without being much moved; it was simply the most available book of his boyhood. He'd also read several cookbooks and was a tolerable cook. There was always a paperback or a pamphlet in his safari jacket or the hip pocket of his khakis. When I'd treated him for snakebite, I'd misinterpreted his intermittent pauses in conversation as lapses into alcoholic stupor.

"No," Shelly said. "His stupor isn't intermittent; it's constant. He was reading the IV bag."

He also had the irritating habit of reading aloud the signs we passed when driving along the highway.

"Mount Olive Baptist Church," he'd say on the road to Flint.

"I beg your pardon."

"That was Mount Olive."

"Oh."

"Welcome to Flint, pop. one-hundred-and-eighteen thousand."

"O.K."

"Days Inn."

"Yes."

Rooster Bootman had warned me that Hack was not immune to dangerously stopping in the middle of a highway if a historical marker caught his eye, and as much as he admired female flesh, he'd read a girl's T-shirt before he noticed her breasts.

Once I saw him inadvertently intimidate four Flint street toughs, staring beyond them at the Ringling Brothers poster on a plate glass window behind the place they loitered. He stood before them, dangling simian arms and squinting balefully as his prognathous jaw worked. The toughs squirmed, becoming visibly unraveled, scattering as Hack moved in to read the finer print.

"Who that mother think he is?" one of the retreating toughs shouted from a safe distance. "Hey, when that corner start belonging to you, man?"

"Do what?" Hack asked me, confused.

"The Greatest Show on Earth."

"Yeah, Barnum and Bailey. What's wrong with them guys?"

"Free-floating anxiety."

"Yeah. Paranoia. It's living in a city does that to people. I wouldn't live in Flint for nothing in the world. Make you crazy as a squirrel in a air raid."

Shelly blamed Hack's parents for his omnivorous appetite for the printed word. His pregnant mother had read aloud to him in the womb, propping Beatrix Potter on her ripe tummy. His father read the entire daily newspaper to Hack until he was three and could read it for himself. According to Tappie Handson, the Grady county librarian, Hack had read virtually every book in the library that he could check out (he wasn't much for hanging around the library) and he read everything in the Grady Junior High School library, including some of the encyclopedias, volumes of which he would take home when he feared a shortage of printed material around his house. "Hack's the stupidest son-of-a-bitch who ever read 20,000 titles," Shelly said. "Tappie and I put a pencil to it once. We figured between road signs, encyclopedias, menus, and catsup bottles, that redneck's read over a billion words."

So I had superficial knowledge of Hack's strange lectophilia before I visited his house and saw his personal library. Shelly had agreed to drop me off at Hack's on her way to the hospital. He'd invited me to "grunt up" some worms to catch shell crackers. The process sounded so outlandish, that I accused him of pulling my leg.

"You cut a wooden stake with an ax, drive a stake in the ground and rub the top of it with the side of the ax blade," he told me. "Red and blue wigglers and sometimes pond worms will just about dance up out the ground."

I asked Shelly if Hack was telling the truth. "He is this time," she snorted.

His house was what a deranged real estate agent might call a "handyman special." It rose like a stained and crooked tooth from a yard infested with weeds and littered with used auto parts. The splotched and weathered boards seemed to creak in the lilting May breeze, but the most conspicuous evidence of life was the dogs. A dozen of them barked, yapped, and howled to herald my arrival. Mongrel dogs, yellow, red, black, and tan, and combinations thereof, scourged under a broken down porch, while pure blooded varieties--pointers, beagles, blueticks, and walkers--hurled themselves against a chain link pen, which was hammered to convexity by their hyperactivity. A gutted '57 Ford rested on concrete blocks. A hubcap filled with rainwater bred mosquito larva on the edge of the worn path to the dangerously dilapidated front steps.

The land behind the house was an actual junkyard, containing goats, fenced in with electrified barbed wire. Multicolored wrecks in various degrees of rust and ruin squatted in motley formation. Sparse tendrils of kudzu wound about them, forming random patches of greenery in areas the goats could not reach. The efficiency of the goats was evidenced not only by the clean patch, but by the surrounding acreage, which was blanketed with the heart-shaped leaves of the advancing Japanese import.

When I'd first come south I'd thought the lush foliage pretty. That was before I knew that it galloped unchecked in southern climes, smothering entire forests. There was an ugly board fence with peeling paint on three sides of my office property. I'd wanted to hide it, cover it with some kind of fast-growing vegetation. I telephoned Miss Ida Worthy about kudzu.

"Kudzu?"

"The vine with the big leaves."

"Yeah, I know what kudzu is, but let me make sure I'm hearing you right," she said. "Did you want to get shed of some kudzu or grow some?"

"I was thinking about covering a fence."

"Well, if you want to get rid of kudzu," she said, "you got to move away and leave it, but if you want to grow some, just drop a cutting and jump the hell back out of the way."

Hack met me at the door. "Hello Doc," he said, "come on in. I'll just put Daddy out, and we can get going." Hack opened a padlocked door and ushered me into a large room, cluttered but clean--orderly in the way a museum that has outgrown its area is orderly. The room was walled with bookshelves which reached to the ceiling. "You can wait here, or you can come with me. I ain't going to be but a minute."

Whose books were these? I was astounded--several thousand volumes, arranged in double rows on the shelves. In the corners magazines, newspapers, and journals were stacked as high as a tall man could reach. This was the testimony to Hack's omnivorous and eccentric scholarship. I knew of his addiction to the printed word, but I never suspected he'd ever read anything of substance, except maybe about reptiles. The subjects here were wide and random. Side by side were books about animal husbandry, a copy of *Moby Dick*, botany lab manuals, *The Cousteau Almanac, White Fang, A Natural History of the Southeastern United States*, as well as *Projectile Points of Tri River Area, The Appalachee Trail, Charlotte's Web, The Complete Poetical Works of Tennyson, Rembrandt's Etchings, The New Mathematics, African Genesis, Sandburg's Lincoln, The Story of O*, and *The Dead Sea Scrolls*. There were also several tables covered with maps, animal bones, arrowheads, butterflies, turtle shells, deer antlers, and mollusk shells.

I knew that Hack was an educator, a principal, but I had viewed his position in the school system as casual, purely administrative and incidental. I figured he was a victim of circumstances in much the same way that I was as I tried to fill the oversized shoes of the village doctor. I had never before thought of him as someone with varied academic interests, someone who had actually read books that were not stapled at the spine. When I met him in the ER, I would have bet money that the pituitary lout with the snakebitten thumb couldn't read the instructions on a matchbook cover. Yet the library that surrounded me, enormous and catholic, testified that the hayseed filling Hack's khakis and brogans surely was far better educated than he seemed.

I heard a pan rattle in the kitchen sink. I followed the noise and found Hack, a wooden toolbox in one hand. His other arm was around a frail white-haired man in overalls. "Come on Daddy," Hack said, "let's put you out."

The old man shuffled across the sloping kitchen floor, his head bobbing mechanically with his dragging feet, *sha, sha, sha*. He reached the screen door, which he let slam behind him as he held the wooden railing and descended the back steps one at a time. Hack unplugged an electric fence transformer and followed the old man to a gate, opened it, and ushered the old man into the junkyard. "Don't let Sarah out," Hack cautioned me as a brown goat walked up, staring with yellow impassive eyes, then nudged me urgently with her horns. "She wants you to scratch her head."

I shut the gate, scratched Sarah's nappy cranium, and followed Hack and his father among the graveyard of abandoned cars and trucks.

"What you working on today, Daddy?" Hack asked the old man, who regarded his son stupidly, his mouth agape. "How about this Impala over here, Daddy? You want to work on this Chevy till dinnertime? O.K., here's your toolbox. I left the metrics in the house cause I figured you'd want to work American today." Hack plugged a 3/4 socket on a ratchet with a 6 inch extender. "Can you say hello to the Doc, Daddy?"

The old man turned to me, his eyes lifeless and his tongue lying thickly in his lower jaw.

"Good morning, Mr. Singletree," I said.

The old man turned stiffly, leaning over the V8 engine, its carburetor topped with an air cleaner the size of a cowboy hat. The hood of the Chevrolet lay on the ground. I noticed that many of the hoods of all the automobiles had been removed, I guessed so that they could not fall on Mr. Singletree in his interminable fugue.

"How long has your father had Alzheimer?" I asked Hack. He closed the gate and plugged in the electric fence.

"Old Timers?" He grinned. "It's been coming on him for a long time, but it got worse after Mamma died in June of 1975."

"You leave him locked in there all day? In an electric fence?"

"He works days in there. He was a mechanic," explained Hack. "He takes things apart, but he can't remember how to get them back together. If he wandered out of the yard, there's no telling what he'd get into. He'll take apart anything he can get next to. He likes cars the best, since that was his work, but he'll tear down your TV, your alarm clock, your fishing reel, anything. Nothing's safe Daddy can get his hands on. He'd take the balls off a brass monkey." Hack closed the gate and fastened it. "I hate it when he wanders up against that fence and it juices him." Hack shook his head. "It's funny, the goats don't forget that fence is hot. They'll try to butt Daddy back if he gets too close, but he remembers that fence better than he remembers anything else. One day he pissed on the bottom strand and it like to have zapped off his tallywacker. Mrs. Green across the road saw what he was fixing to do before he done it and yelled at him to stop, but he went ahead on. She said it knocked him off his feet and rolled him like a syrup bucket, with him hollering and pissing himself and rolling on the ground. She said there's one thing Daddy ain't forgot how to do and that's cuss. She said the goats ran every which way, scrambling up on the cars." Hack paused, watching his daddy at work on the Chevrolet. "I know its a shame to pasture out your own daddy, Doc, but damn if I can think of another thing in the wide world to do. He'll ride in the truck, but he don't like to stay in the house and watch T.V. He'll climb in one of the cars if it gets to raining. May's cafe brings him his dinner." He smiled wistfully, "Boy, didn't I have a time getting his hair to lay back down after he pissed on that wire."

"He needs to be in an institution," I said softly, "where he can be cared for."

"What institution?" said Hack. "Not Lilies of the Field Nursing Home. I wouldn't put my redbone hound in that place. I damn sure ain't putting my own daddy over yonder. Mamma made me swear I wouldn't anyway."

The nursing home, owned by the Wrights and operated by Beulah and Lee Bob Parker, was a prime and shameful example of unregulated free enterprise in the health care business. The facility kept its overhead down and its profits up by staffing with untrained, minimum wage misfits and goons, who generally enjoyed dominion over the aged and infirm. Old folks with walkers or wheelchairs wandered the halls immodestly dressed and unsupervised while orderlies flirted with practical nurses or watched television in the day room. The air was permeated with an overpowering odor of urine and cherry disinfectant. The building should have been condemned.

Besides the goats, a tremendous sow shuffled around among the abandoned cars.

"Is that my pig Syndrome over there?" I asked.

Hack smiled, "It shore is, and she's a good sow too for keeping the snakes down so Daddy don't get bit. Melvin stuck her in there when she got too big for his dog pen."

I'd received the pig as payment for treating Hollis Rhodes' arthritis. I was supposed to have her butchered for my fee but found I didn't have the heart, so I asked Melvin Dryden to keep her, since I owed him money for his perpetual repair bill on my car. Pigs were reputed to hunt poisonous snakes, skin them by pawing with their sharp hooves, and eat them. They were supposed to be immune to snake venom, but Hack told me that it was more likely that the snakes' fangs couldn't penetrate the tough hide and layer of fat to reach the muscle where the hemotoxin can do more damage.

"Sure hogs eat rattlesnakes," he affirmed. "They eat anything they get a holt of. They'll eat their own piglets. They'll eat a man."

"What?"

"You heard about the man who took drunk and the hogs ate him?"

"I thought that was a joke."

"Naw. They'll eat you first chance they get. Hogs ate Harry Walden, but mostly when hogs eat somebody, it's somebody who's dropped dead in the hog pen of a heart attack or a stroke, but you got to be real careful to keep your younguns away from hogs. 'Course Syndrome there's a right civilized sow. I taught her to fetch, roll over, and speak. She'll eat a rattlesnake, though. I come home one evening and found Daddy treed up on a Buick. Syndrome had about a four-foot timber rattler in her mouth, swinging her head and slapping that snake first one side of her belly and then the other. She ate that snake like a noodle."

I followed him to a shed, where he found an ax, a board, and a tomato can, then we walked around the house to a rough garden whose only spring growth had volunteered from the summer before. He sharpened the board on one end. "Well, here we go," he said. "You hold her while I drive her in."

"Is a board what you use to grunt the worms with?"

"Yep, unless you want to use it to stab a vampire. Hold her steady now, so I don't bust up them precious hands."

I held the stake, cringing and looking away as Hack used the blunt end of the ax to pound the stake deep into the ground. "Don't be so nervous, Doc. I ain't liable to hit your hand or your head either one. I done this one time before, back when I was a teenager."

Hack's overhead swing repeatedly struck the stake, which vibrated and mushroomed under his ax. Suddenly he paled, stopping to catch his breath, leaning on his ax helve and rubbing his arm.

"Hurt your arm?"

"Naw, I just jarred my crazybone."

"Ever feel any pain in your jaw?"

"Yeah, when I win second place in a fistfight. Well, that's good enough anyway."

"How about pressure or tightness in your chest?"

"Quit playing doctor and pay attention." Hack squatted in front of the stake. Holding the blade and the upper helve, he rubbed the side of the ax head on the top of the stake, making sounds like, well, grunts, which brought Syndrome as close to us as the electric fence would allow. "It works on hogs," I observed.

Then next to the heel of Hack's brogan, the glossy caramel tip of an earthworm appeared. I took it between my thumb and index finger and tried to pull it out of the ground. It stretched until I thought it would break but wouldn't come. Hack resumed grunting and the worm slipped easily out of the ground. I dropped it into the tomato can and noticed the appearance of others, which I quickly collected.

Having harvested our bait, we drove to a pond where Hack knew the shellcrackers were bedding. He said he could *smell out* the beds. As he paddled a wooden skiff into the shallow water where a creek fed the pond, I was surprised that I could detect the fishy aroma of the bedding grounds too, but I didn't see how we could catch fish in water that was no more than a foot-and-a-half deep. "Shhh," he said, easing down the concrete block he used as an anchor, "you'll spook them." He instructed me to bait my hook and pitch it near the edge of a clear area composed of a number of shallow craters on the sandy bottom.

"Hook the worm once through the clitellum?" I whispered, indicating the beige ring around a pond worm.

"Yeah, you can hook it once through the clitellum or you can hook it twice through the ass. The fish ain't particular when they're on a bed. The males are keeping the beds clean. When one carries your worm off the nest, you hook *him* in the lip and throw his ass in the cooler."

The instant I dropped my worm into the water, the cork began to move slowly without going under. "Pull him now," Hack said. I did and hooked a fish that bent my telescopic pole double and made my monofilament line sing. The fish was of the variety northerners called panfish. This one had golden scales and a scarlet quarter moon of crimson color at the edge of its gill cover. It was wider than Hack's hand. He had to hold it against his chest to remove the hook.

"A titty bream," he announced, grinning. "You're always wondering how to tell the sexes apart," he said, squeezing the fish, which spurted a thin stream of liquid half the length of the skiff. "Here's a male. The earthworm you hooked in the clitellum is a hermaphrodite, which is able to hook up in reciprocal fertilization with another earthworm. Me, I'm a mature heterosexual male, who's gone wash the worm-goo and fish-slime off his hands as soon as we get done angling and go over to the Magnolia Motel and knock him off a piece of prime U.S. grade-A ass from a mature heterosexual female."

"Are you going to meet Beulah?"

Hack's jaw dropped. "What do you know about Beulah?"

The fish bit regularly and slowly, the cork hardly moving at all. I caught shellcrackers as fast as I could take one off and re-bait the hook, but Hack stopped me after about a dozen.

"That's enough of them," he said. "Let's run over to your place and catch a bass before we call it a morning."

Chapter Fifteen

I was paddling Hack around in the jonboat he kept on Loonie Lake. We were fishing for largemouth bass. Since his snakebite, he'd shared the fish he caught in my backyard and offered me the use of his boat, but he'd made no arrangements to pay his bill. When he invited me to go fishing in Lake Loonie (as though it were his property), he'd decided rather than having to keep me in fish, he'd leave me an old baitcaster and some gummy plastic worms. "Just ease us up to that grassy point and cast to the bank, Doc," he said. "That's where they hang around before they go on the bed." It was a beautiful May morning. The woods around the lake were full of bright greenery. The sun warmed our faces and sparkled the water.

"Most folks fish a worm too fast," Hack said grinning. "But not you." My worm lay comatose on the bottom while I picked at a backlash that looked like a jaybird nest. "You take your time." The water was lapping the throat of the metal bow.

"You got to ease it along like so, raising the tip of your rod and taking up the slack, till you feel her bump it." After a somewhat long pause, Hack said, "I've got a confession to make, Doc."

I watched his floating line start moving away in jerking motions. "You've got a bite!"

"Hush. She'll get it in her mouth and start swimming away. You watch the line tighten . . . ." He leaned forward, holding his rod with both hands and bracing one brogan against the gunwale. "You take up the slack . . . ." He slowly turned the handle of the reel. "Then . . . you . . . get ready . . . to HAIR-LIP her! Hard!"

His rod bent double and quivered. The line tightened and stretched, slinging bright waterbeads into the sunlight. The fish made a run, taking drag, and Hack hollered, "Yah hoo!" The bass broke the surface, lashing the water into lace and leaping high, shaking, rattling its gills. As he brought the fish nearer the boat, I could see its white sides flashing gold in the brown water. When he wrestled it to the surface, he caught it by its lower lip, holding up a bass with a mouth large enough to bite a grapefruit. It was a trophy fish he estimated would weigh nine or ten pounds--bronze-backed and silver with a broken pewter line down its side and bright red gills. "Well, here's supper for you and Shelly both. I've got the shellcrackers promised to a friend who flat loves to eat a mess of bream. In fact, it's the second to best thing she likes to do."

He removed the hook and strung the fish, handing me the cord. I tied it to the stern and headed in. Hack wasn't a man to catch more fish than he needed. The big bass made one run against the stringer, yawing the boat. Hack laughed, "If we can get the lady to gee-haw, you won't have to paddle." *Gee* and *haw*, I'd learned, were the directional signals given to mules when plowing.

"How'd you know it was a female?" I asked as we beached the boat. More of the gender theme.

"The way she wiggled her hips," he said fanning his hands in the air.

We'd had this conversation before. He'd said the same thing about sexing rattlesnakes, a remark which sent Shelly storming out of the ER. The gender question had become a common theme in our chats. He readily discriminated the sexes of animals, and he treated females as a different species entirely, a quality I had first attributed to sexism. I soon learned that as a woodsman, he was primarily interested in animal behavior, not sexist conclusions, but Shelly insisted that he was chauvinistic in his attitude toward women too, that he also treated female human beings as a species apart.

"You said *her* before you set the hook."

He pinched a clot of Redman chewing tobacco from its paper pouch, shook off the loose ends, and set the wad in the side of his jaw. "I was fishing for sow-bass," he mumbled. "They're bigger. I figured the females would be biting. It's time for them to go on the bed, and they're feeding fast for the extra protein they need for making eggs." His speech improved as he organized the lump in his cheek. "All the girls, from mosquitoes to debutantes, frenzy feed in the name of motherhood. This one here's already full of roe. See how her belly's swole?"

"Can you eat the roe?" I thought of caviar. I hadn't tasted caviar since I'd become a transplanted Southerner.

"Yeah, mix it up with scrambled eggs. Uh, like I told you before we tied into the bass, I've got a minor confession to make."

"What is it you wish to confess, my son?"

He laughed, wiping the corner of his mouth. "I'm pretty sure I know who Gatorman is," he said.

"You don't say."

"It's a fellow named Potter Fish Kinnard, an Indian half breed, who lives on Mulgrove Ridge in the Toa. We were between his cabin and the Capachequi when we saw his tracks."

I was wary. Shelly had just about convinced me that the Gatorman was Hack's hoax. "Why didn't we go on to his cabin?" I asked. "Why didn't we follow his footprints?"

He raised his eyebrows, turned his head, and spit into the water. Minnows attacked the dark brown spittle, breaking it up. "Which question you want me to answer first?"

"Why didn't we follow the footprints to his cabin?"

"All the tracks headed *away* from his cabin. There were three sets of footprints of the same man. They were all aimed toward the Capachequi. There's four mounds in there 120 feet above sea level, which means they rise out of the swamp about 80 feet."

"How could three sets of footprints of the same person be going the same direction?"

"He was walking in a circle, going somewhere, likely to the mounds, and coming back another way."

"Why would he do that?"

"So nobody could see what he was dragging."

"Which was?"

"Corn malt."

"How do you know it wasn't a tail?"

"I found a sprouted kernel of corn in the drag marks, and the croaker printed the mud."

"Croaker?"

"Burlap sack. Besides, Kinnard ain't got a tail."

"Why would he care if anybody saw him carrying corn?"

"There's only two things you can do with corn in the swamp, and neither one of them's legal. A man don't want to be seen hauling corn into a swamp."

"O.K. Sherlock, Kinnard is either making whiskey or baiting deer, right?" I was proud of my deduction.

"He's making whiskey, Watson."

"You're sure?"

"I'm dead sure. Kinnard don't have to bait deer to kill as many as he wants. If he did, he wouldn't bait them away from his cabin just to kill one and drag it a mile. He's having enough trouble dragging thirty pounds of corn malt. He's hauling it in, then coming back along the ridge, probably after dark. He's sick, or he'd be toting the corn on his back."

"How old is Kinnard?

"I don't know. Seventy-five or eighty. He's about Daddy's age."

"Maybe he's just old."

"Well, he's sick too. You remember that smell we couldn't place? It was garlic for one thing. He's probably wearing garlic around his neck and a sachet. There ain't no telling what all's in that sachet."

"Do sick people wear garlic around their neck?"

"Yep."

"What kind of sick?"

"Lots of things. Colds, high blood. They eat it for worms, liver, gallbladder, snakebite. You ought to know. Most blacks around here have high blood. You're the doctor."

"I thought you said he was an Indian, a Native American."

Hack grinned. "He's a Indian all right, 'cause that's what he says he is. Which ain't to argue he don't have some black blood too. We ain't talking pedigrees and bird dogs, Doc. They probably ain't been no pure-blooded humans since Neanderthal Man."

"I haven't ordered patients to wear garlic garlands for a while, but if it was garlic, why didn't we recognize it?"

"We weren't expecting it. And whatever else was in his sachet bag was probably mixed up with asafetida."

"Which is . . . ?"

"A high smelling root sap, called *devil's dung* and *food for the gods*, depending on your point of view. It's used for a carminative."

"To cause flatulence?"

"Yep, farting. It's also used as an antispasmodic. Then Kinnard was leaking off a *sick* smell too. Then there was the malt. There was enough stink around those tracks to baffle a bloodhound. On top of all that, me and you were drinking whiskey, which brings us back around to another reason we didn't follow the smell or the tracks on into the swamp."

"We didn't follow him because you didn't want to walk up on his still."

"It shows a lack of breeding, yeah."

"And we could have gotten shot, right?"

"It's possible. Bad manners has got more than one snooper shot in Grady County."

"Well, how big is Kinnard? Does he weigh 300 pounds, like the creature who left the footprints?" I thought I'd caught him in a mistake. His deductions, however clever, didn't explain the strangely distorted footprints with their claw marks in the mud.

"Not the last time I saw him. That was about five years ago when I was hog hunting the ridge. Kinnard's about my size, or was."

"Do you mean he may be transformed in some way," I smiled.

"Yeah Doc, and he may've changed some too," Hack grinned. "If it's him leaving them footprints, it ain't like the same Indian I used to know. Who wouldn't leave no footprints a-tall. Not near his still or around a bushhook he'd robbed. If it's Fish Kinnard, something bad's wrong with him."

We dragged the jonboat up on the shore and took the tackle and fish to the house. He swung the bass into the kitchen sink. Taking a flask out from his pocket, he sprinkled some moonshine into the fish's gills. "For flavor," he said with a wink.

"We're not going to eat the gills."

"You wait and see," he said. "That little bit of stump will flavor the whole fish. The gills will spread it through her, just like oxygen. Get me a sharp knife and let me show you how to clean a bass."

I watched as he made a slash behind the gills and cut alongside the dorsal fin. Deftly guiding his knife around the ribs, he sliced off a thick fillet, which he skinned in one quick motion exposing pearly flesh. Then he removed two bright yellow and grainy lobes of roe and put them in a saucer. "You do the other side." He turned the bass over and presented it to me.

"Nothing to it," I bragged. "I'll just make a posterior to anterior incision from the dorsal fin to the vertebral body, then make a blunt dissection around the ribs." I filleted the fish.

"Well, I'll be dipped," Hack said. "Looks like you learned one thing worth a damn in med school after all. You did better than me." He spit into the drain and chased down the tobacco by turning on the faucet.

Insisting that "the sweetest meat is closest to the bone," he severed the backbone from the head and included it in the pan with the fillets. "Which is why we court skinny girls," he added, "along with the robust ones." I'd learned that Hack's brand of chauvinism bore no malice. He considered the females of the species biologically superior to the male--prettier, smarter, able to endure more pain. He flirted shamelessly with all women, young, old, married, single, seductive, or plain and felt it poor manners not to acknowledge in every transaction with the female gender the magnetism of opposite flesh, which he considered the sexual mandates of his biological duty.

Most women except Shelly smiled when he came around, even though he wasn't one to labor for political correctness. "Well, Miss Shelly," he'd said one day in the form of a greeting. "I shore do like the way you fill up a pair of britches." He'd seemed genuinely puzzled by the vehemence of her response. "What's got all the girls upset?" he asked. "It's the same way with the teachers over at the junior high, so it must be the gibbus moon. It's just like when you keep a bunch of heifers, they all come in season at once."

"I think they just want to be treated equally, the same way you treat men," I had said, hoping Shelly was out of earshot of the heifer hypothesis.

"If you believe that," he'd said, astounded, "you a bigger fool than I thought."

I walked him to his truck. I wanted to ask him another question or two about the Gatorman before he set out for the Magnolia Motel with his cooler of shellcrackers, his wampum.

"A while ago you said that garlic was used to treat high blood. Is high blood the same as hypertension?"

"There you go. Weak blood is anemia, and bad blood is syphilis. Just plain blood is kin. Doc, you about to get yourself on the right track."

"Does Kinnard live alone in the swamp?"

"Yep, his land is smack in the middle of Toa Plantation. Kinnard hunts, traps, and runs trotlines. His whiskey still's probably on one of the mounds in the Capachequi so the spring rains won't flood him out. A branch runs along those mounds that Kinnard can use to cool his worm during the dry season. He'd have to go out there by skiff when the water table's up."

"His worm?"

"His coil. His condenser, he's got to cool his condenser with water. You ain't made much whiskey, have you Doc?"

"Not much, no."

"You got to cool your worm." He winked.

"I've distilled water."

"O.K., it's the same thing, except you start off with malt beer instead of water. Some people think the part of the Toa we found Kinnard's footprints is near the seven villages of the Capachequi in DeSoto's journals," Hack continued. "I think it's the place. Kinnard don't come out of there much. His folks didn't either. There used to be a lot of Indians around here. Kinnard's granddaddy or great granddaddy was a runaway slave that the Creeks took in and protected, made him an official member of the tribe and let him marry a squaw before white settlers run most of the Indians off in the 1830's. They didn't run Kinnard's great granddaddy off on account of his African blood or maybe on account that none of the Kinnards fought on the wrong side in the Battle of Chicasawhatchee in 1836. You was better off being black in those days than Indian if you wanted to own land in Grady County."

I was medically interested in Kinnard's mysterious transformation. If Hack's estimation of the old man's weight were accurate, he had gained close to one-hundred pounds. I had seen his footprints myself which indicated extreme swelling of the feet, some kind of elephantiasis or edema. "When are you game to go back in there?" I asked.

"The water table's up. We'll go in from the high side. If we go out late this afternoon, after you get off work and I get off my little project, we can catch Chief Potter Fish Kinnard on the roost. He'll come home at duskdark. A sick Indian's got better sense than to wander around the Toa after dark. Even if a Yankee and a redneck ain't. I'll be back later this evening." He cranked his truck, which protested, then caught. It emitted a blanket of thick smoke.

Hack stuck his head out the window. "Melvin Dryden can't make this sumbitch quit smoking, but he says I can put some citronella in the gas tank and fog mosquitoes."

"Thanks for the fish."

"Any time."

"Say hello to Beulah for me."

71

"I don't expect I'll get around to that."

Chapter Sixteen

Hack's truck disappeared, leaving a layer of blue smoke hovering in the late morning air. Shelly came for lunch, and I broiled the fish fillets in butter and parsley. They retained a hint of whiskey that the gills' final gasps carried into the flesh. Shelly loved it. She asked if it came from Loonie Lake, and I told her it did. I neglected to tell her Hack caught it. I didn't want to spoil her lunch.

She dropped me off at the hospital to look in on the patients. Then I went by the pharmacy to draw a couple of syringes of Lasix and Digoxin and to pick up Digoxin, Lasix, and Hydralazine tablets. The more I thought about it, the surer I was that Kinnard suffered from congestive heart failure that resulted in diffuse edema, swelling of lower extremities, caused, perhaps, by long standing hypertension and subsequent hypertensive cardiomyopathy. In other words, he was bloated up from retention of body fluids. I put the syringes, the tablets, my stethoscope, some antibiotics, and a BP cuff in my ruck sack, which was actually a WWII gas mask pack I'd bought for $1.50 at Top Sarge, an Army Surplus store in East Flint. The bag was just the ticket for carrying my notebook, a camera, and a peanut butter sandwich on my orientation outings. Shelly was on duty tonight, so I didn't have to worry about being late.

As I was getting ready to leave the hospital with Buster, who agreed to drive me home, Margaret Holt stopped me. "Where you goin' with them syringes, Doctor?"

"I'm making a house call to the residence of a gentleman named Potter Fish Kinnard, whom I suspect of having congestive heart failure."

"Ha! You making a shack call, is what you making."

"Anyway, that's where I'm headed with these syringes."

"Well, take you a flack jacket in case you catch him drunk and some Valium in case you catch him sober. He'll be one way or the other if he true to form."

"Mrs. Holt, everybody is either drunk or sober or somewhere in between."

"Well, he'll be drunk or somewhere in between."

"He imbibes, does he?"

"Naw, he guzzles!"

"Anything else?"

"I guess you taking some diuretic, since you say he endemic."

"I didn't say he was endemic."

"If he got congestive heart disease, he endemic."

"I was just going for a diuretic now."

"And two tourniquets, don't forget them."

"Tourniquets, what do I want with tourniquets?"

"For when he cuts Hack Singletree with his razor and shoots you with his twelve gauge for trespassing down there. He don't stay out yonder to make no new Yankee friends."

"Thank you, Mrs. Holt," I said, leaving. What made me think she didn't hold me in her highest regard? I paused in the doorway, "How did you know I was going with Hack Singletree?"

"Well, ain't you?"

"Yes."

"That's what I thought. You ain't got *much* business in that swamp a-tall, and you ain't got *no* business in there by yourself."

Hack and I entered the swamp from the south side, driving for an hour on county roads and another thirty minutes on roads with names like Lonesome, Hardup, Cheehaw, and Muskogee; until finally, after many nameless red dirt lanes fronting the most abject poverty I had ever seen, we turned off on what was nothing more than two trails with a grass median connecting a series of mud holes.

"This road used to have three trails when I was a kid," Hack said. "A lot of the dirt roads did."

"Why?"

"For one-horse wagons and buckboards. The wagon wheels made two trails and the horse made one in the middle."

Finally we stopped. "Here's the ridge," Hack said. "We'll hike a ways down that path yonder, and I'll introduce you to the illustrious Potter Fish Kinnard." We followed a twisted path along the ridge until we came to a cornfield that was hand-picked and abandoned since last summer. Mourning doves cooed in the early evening air and bobwhites whistled, calling to their mates. I noticed that the corn was overgrown with weeds, that vines with blue flowers entwined the dry stalks that whispered in the light spring breeze.

The pine trees along the ridge were much larger than any I had ever seen. Tall and straight with thick shingles of mauve bark; some of them must have been six feet in circumference. "Virgin timber," Hack explained. "These woods have never been cut over, not the pine, the oak, or the cypress. Those pines are several hundred years old. Kinnard owns the most valuable timber per acre in Georgia, but he won't cut it. He ain't got a pot to piss in, but he still won't cut his timber. Not many folks understand that, but I do. Kinnard can't even pay the taxes. Mr. Mack--that's Robert McCormick Jones--pays the taxes for him, but that ain't common knowledge, so don't tell it around."

"Why would Jones do that?"

74

Hack grinned. "Why does a buzzard fly, a frog hop, and a polecat lick his ass?"

"Why?"

"Because they *can*."

"Oh."

"Like I told you before we came, Jones owns Toa Plantation. He's a conservationist. He likes having a wild Indian running around in yonder to keep paleface poachers out. About thirty thousand acres of the plantation is wetlands, which Jones lets Kinnard have the run of, but he don't let nobody else go in there."

"Except you?"

"Uh, except me. Mr. Mack's got the idea that the Toa Swamp complex is crucial to the hydro-ecology of the entire southwest portion of the state, the southeast portion of Alabama, and the Florida Panhandle."

"Is that possible?"

"Hell yes. He's right."

"Couldn't he acquire Kinnard's land by paying the taxes?"

"Sure, but like I said, he's a conservationist, and that means conserving Kinnard, who's the wildest thing in the Toa. Jones likes Kinnard's reverence for the swamp, which is a holy place to him, but Jones ain't no fool. I expect he's made some deal with Kinnard to keep Kinnard's chunk of Toa from going to the pulpwood and paper companies, since Kinnard's got no heirs. He probably got Kinnard to sign a quit claim, which Kinnard might do since he trusts Mr. Mack and he don't trust hardly nobody else. Jones figures if everybody leaves the swamp alone, it'll someday look like Kinnard's chunk of it, this part you're in now."

"Will it?"

"Well, it'll look pretty good in a hundred years."

The high part of Jones' Toa Plantation, according to Hack, was wiregrass and longleaf pine. It was farmed in narrow strips to provide protection and habitat for the wildlife. Toa Plantation, which resembled Georgia farmland in the '30s, was being converted into an ecological research center directed by Lindwood Honer, a scientist with a Ph.D. in forestry. Honer's wife Katrina was a wetlands specialist. Together with a team of resident scientists they were trying to learn how to use the land in best accord with its conservation.

"They're good folks with the right idea," Hack said, "none of the usual bullshit about how our research will show how we can save the forests and wetlands, but we got to cut the timber and drain the swamp for money to fund it. They got about as good a stand of longleaf pine there is left in Georgia, and they're out to conserve it and to learn better ways of land and water conservation, period. They don't have to answer to nobody but Mr. Mack and the foundation while they're doing it."

"What's so rare about pine trees in Georgia? They're everywhere. Like churches in Spain."

Hack stopped dead in his tracks. "I'm talking about *native* Georgia pine trees, Doc, not that shit you see in rows that grows like a weed and won't outlive a bulldog. I ain't talking about slash pine and loblolly. I'm talking about a goddamn tree that grows up slow and straight and tall and lives five or six centuries if lightning don't strike it or if some dickhead don't flick a match or saw it down for a telephone pole. I'm talking about a tree whose needles whisper and hiss in the wind, that grow so straight and tall you fall over backwards and bust you ass when you look at the top."

"The big trees you called virgins a minute ago?"

"That's right. *Hell* yes. Those are longleaf pine trees that were already here when that swineherd DeSoto came through with his army, torturing Indians and looking for gold. One or two of them was probably here when Columbus set his Italian ass on the continent." Hack's hostility toward outsiders made me think he might have Native American blood himself.

"Is the research center the outfit citizens are protesting for closing off 17 miles of the Tsallahatchee Creek?"

"Yeah, but if the Tsallahatchee had been under the stewardship of those *concerned* citizens over yonder, they'd of turned it into a dump for old air conditioners, batteries, and junkyard cars. One of those *concerned* citizens has been shocking up catfish with an old crank telephone. He's pissed because the Department of Natural Resources patrols the creek better than they used to, but he's a trespasser. They all are. That creek's been on private property since before the War Between the States."

"Where's all this money coming from?"

"Jones."

We walked beneath gigantic live oaks, whose heavy branches sagged nearly to the ground, branches that were wide enough for a man to walk upon. The high canopy of oaks and other trees blocked out the sun so that there was little underbrush except for a few palmettoes and Spanish bayonets. The land dropped off sharply, and at the bottom of the ridge the cypress forest began, the enormous bases of the celery-shaped trunks wider than a man's armspan, their stalagmite roots taller than I was. The area was dark, strange, enchanted. "I've got only one more question," I announced.

"What's that?"

"Shouldn't we be afraid of the Indian?"

"Not now."

76

"No?"

"We ain't down there yet."

The deeper we went into the forest, the quieter we got until we came to a rough log cabin, patched by salvaged signs, boxes, and burlap bags. The cabin squatted on fossiliforus limestone boulders. Nearby was a padlocked shed next to a makeshift wire fence that held a hog and two goats. Some chickens, a few inside the fence, the others out, pecked and scratched.

"He wouldn't shoot us, would he?" I asked timidly.

"That depends."

"On what?"

"On how blind he is, or how drunk. He used to be a friend of Daddy's, so he knows me. 'Course he ain't got the least reason not to shoot *you*. In the old days, he wouldn't shoot. He'd just slip up on you, slit your throat, and pull your tongue out through the hole. Then maybe he'd ask you what you wanted and how could he help you."

A pileated woodpecker knocked its hollow head against a longleaf pine, and a blue jay squawked loudly from a sweetgum. "Chief Fish!" Hack called. "Youuu, Fish Kinnard!" Hack had his hands open and out to his sides.

The bluejay screamed this time. We waited. "It's Singletree!" Hack shouted, "I want to come up there!" We walked carefully up the creaking plank steps. The weathered gray door was missing a knob. In its place was a hole bisected by a greasy horsehair string that hung across the inside of the hole. "He's home," said Hack, "or his latch string would be hanging out the hole. Chief, I want to come on in there, and there's another fellow, a white doctor, here with me. I'm gone reach through the door hole now and pull the latch string if that's aw right with you." I heard an animal sound, a wheezing followed by a rumble and a growl or a raspy cough.

"What was that?" I said.

"Hold your hands out to the side," Hack said. "I hope that was Kinnard saying come ahead on."

Hack reached into the doorknob hole, hooked the string with his index finger, and pulled it until I heard a wooden click of a latch being lifted. Then he pushed the door open. A slice of twilight fell along the wide gray planks of the floor, illuminating a shapeless form which seemed somehow alive without being human. As my eyes and mind strained to assimilate the creature folded into the corner, I was assaulted by an overwhelming odor, powerful and fetid yet tinged with garlic and wood smoke. Utterances I could distinguish as human but not understand issued from the lump in the dark corner. As my eyes adjusted to the dim light, I moved forward, noticing misshapen wet footprints leading across the wide plank floor toward the sounds.

"Mr. Kinnard?"

The bundle wrapped in blankets and burlap moved forward, and the light transected a human visage so severe that I gasped and jerked backward. The old man's face was more reptilian than human, lined with deep creases like twisted naugahyde spread over wide cheekbones and centered by a blade of a nose. A splinter of that light fell on a clouded eye, and I shuddered. I edged closer to discover that the strange and incomprehensible shapes resting on a wood box padded in deerskin were two human feet and ankles swollen to monstrous proportions and seeping fluid. His curved toenails were black and flinty and six to eight inches long. There was no way he could reach them to keep them trimmed. I had expected edema, but this was by far the worst case I'd ever seen. Kinnard's legs were like elephant legs. He had cut his overalls up the seams to allow for the tumescent flesh. The entire lower part of his body, his abdomen, his legs, and his feet, was as inflated with liquid as a wine skin.

"Open some windows, Hack. Let's get some light and air in here." Kinnard's back was propped up by a feed sack. He probably couldn't lie down without accumulating fluids in his lungs, so he had to sleep sitting up.

"Well, Hack," said a gravelly voice. "You say you brung a friend? Hit's a coons age since you come to the Toa. Git you a drink." There was a plastic milk jug on the kitchen table with some jelly glasses and some small ceramic cups. Hack poured into three of the cups.

"Nothing for me," I said. "I'm working, and Mr. Kinnard shouldn't have any either."

Hack ignored me, handing out the moonshine. The old man's head jutted out from his burlap hood. The hair was nappy and white as dirty cotton, pulled back into a blunt pony tail, and the eyes were cloudy with cataracts. "Erkawhack, whack, whack," he coughed. Veins swollen by the pressure of backed up fluids bulged in his neck. A gnarled hand reached out for the cup, fumbling until Hack took the wrist and nestled the ceramic cup into his fingers. The cloudy eyes watered.

"I figured you'd be drunk, Chief," said Hack.

The old man managed a rasping laugh. "I cain't handle him like I used to," he said. "I finally catch up. Now I kin make him faster than I kin drink him up, and I done got right damn slow makin' him too."

"Well, this stuff here's pretty good," Hack said. "I'd say it's as good as any you ever built."

Kinnard grinned, toothless and vague. "I don't jump up and down good as I used to, and I've done got blind. But how's your daddy doing? What's old Elroy Singletree been up to? He ain't dead?"

"Naw, he's fine, Chief. He's done got old too, mean as a blacksnake, and forgetful, but he's getting long aw right. Say, what you doing all swole up?"

"Hit's the dropsy, Hack. Couldn't find me no foxglove. Say, you ain't seen none, has you? Used to be all about an around here, but I be damned if I kin find air bit when it's a use."

"I ain't seen none, but maybe the Doc here's got something will juice you up."

"Horseradish heps me sometime," said Kinnard.

"What's foxglove?" I asked Hack.

"A flower with little bell-shaped blossoms. You've heard of digitalis. He'd make him a tea to slow his heart rate down and get himself to pissing like a cripple coon. Folks take it for dropsy, which is what the chief's got, wouldn't you say."

"I'd like to listen to his heart and take his blood pressure before I make a diagnosis, but it does look like congestive heart failure, yes."

"This here is Dr. Otis Stone, Chief. He wants to listen to yore heart."

"You mean he cain't hear it from over there where he's at? I kin damn shore hear that sumbitch. Hit sound like a wet mop slapping up side the house." The old man reached out blindly with his hand, which I took in mine. The palms and fingers were callused and dry, the skin cool as a lizard's.

I attached the blood pressure cuff and pumped it up. Kinnard had a BP of 220/120 and a heart rate of 120. I took his temperature. When I unbuttoned his shirt and listened with the stethoscope, his heart sounded like the William Tell Overture--Da-Da-Dump, Da-Da-Dump--the classic gallup rhythm--and his lungs crackled like cellophane as the alveoli popped open and wheezed as air tried to escape through the engorged and narrowed bronchial tubes. Hack wanted to listen, and I let him while I gave Kinnard an 0.5 mg injection of digoxin and 40 mg of Lasix. I'd follow up with .25 mg of digoxin in six hours along with another 40 of Lasix. After twelve hours I'd do the same thing again. We were going to spend the night in the swamp.

Chapter Seventeen

Kinnard suffered from malignant hypertension; his heart muscle, after years of pumping against the high pressure in his arteries, was on the downward slope of Starling's curve--his failing heart had dilated beyond cardiac efficiency and his heart valves had started leaking.

"You sound like breakfast, Chief," Hack said. "Your lungs got the snap, crackle, pop of Rice Crispies, and your ticker sounds like a pot of boiling grits."

Kinnard wanted to hear. He grinned weakly as he listened to the stethoscope. "You wrong, Hack. The crackling is the fire of my spirit burning to be free."

"Naw it ain't, Chief. The doc here is about to see to it you got plenty moons left. If that's a fire in yonder he's fixing to put it out."

I asked Hack if he could heat some water and bring in the washtub I'd seen hanging on the outside wall of the cabin. I wanted to soak Kinnard's feet and trim the talons that grew where his toenails should have been. Besides being caked with black swamp mud, the thick toes were crusted with fluids that seeped through his cracked skin and dried.

"Is there anything around here I can use to cut your toenails, Mr. Kinnard?"

"I bet he ain't got no boltcutters," said Hack, who was building a fire in the wood stove and lighting kerosene lamps now that the sun was fully down.

"What have you been eating, Mr. Kinnard? What can we fix for your supper?"

"Bull yearling soup," the old man said. "Since my stomach gone bad, all I eat is bull yearling soup. I cain't get around good enough to get up much else."

"What's bull yearling soup?" I asked Hack.

He thought about it, scratching his whiskers. "Beats me," he finally said.

"What you say you been eating, Chief?" Hack said. "Tell me where it is and I'll fix some up for you."

"Bull yearling soup," he repeated. "Up over the stove."

Hack laughed, "Bouillon is what he means. And lordy ain't he got a bunch of it?" On the shelf over the stove were jar after jar of chicken and beef bouillon cubes wrapped in silver and gold foil.

"Don't fix him that," I said. "That stuff's pure sodium. That's one reason he's retaining all that fluid."

"There's nothing else here," said Hack.

"They ain't nothing else here 'cause I can't eat nothing else," Kinnard complained.

"Where's your chickens roost, Chief? Could you eat some chicken if I hem one up."

"You cotch him and bile him up, I kin eat him or drink him one. He got so he

80

about wear me out to cotch him, and I can't see to bust his ass down with the doublebarrel or find them eggs. They roost out yonder in one them trees or tother and build them nests got-knows-where off in them damn briars," the old man smiled, his nose resting on his chin.

"You ain't been able to find a bushhook or trotline and get you a catfish?" Hank teased.

"I don't rob no sethooks," the old man snapped.

Hack grinned and went outside, and I knelt beside the steaming washtub where Kinnard soaked his feet. I washed them gently with a surgical sponge from the canvas pack. Hack had found some pruning shears Kinnard used on his scuppernongs.

Overcoming the initial revulsion of sight and smell, one by one I clipped the thick nails in the light of the kerosene lantern, listening to the whip-poor-wills' plaintive call and the deep and occasional drum of a bullfrog from the thick darkness of the swamp. Later I would remember that pure moment and return to it during times of personal and professional confusion. Unencumbered by expensive equipment, nurses, insurance waivers, sterile hospital sheets, and malpractice suits, I was a healer, purely and simply caring for his patient with concern and confidence in that time honored bond between the medicine man and the infirm, while chickens screamed and squawked hysterically outside, drowning out the other night sounds.

"There you are, Mr. Kinnard. I believe you'll be able to get around better."

"I warrant I will, Dr. Stone, and I'm much obliged for a service I ain't liable to forget."

I walked out to the dilapidated porch to see if I could help Hack. "Come hold the lantern!" he hollered. He held a young rooster upside down by its legs.

In the lamplight, the chicken was the rich orange and gold of burnished copper and bronze. Its yellow eyes, confused by the light, blinked, and the bright comb shook as the head jerked around bewildered.

I took the lantern. With one hand, Hack picked up an ax at the balancing point of the helve. With the other he rested the rooster's neck on a cylindrical section of sawed log used as a chopping block. The rooster cocked his head, blinking his eyes as Hack raised the ax and let it drop. The decapitated bird beat its furious wings with violent finality, spurting blood from the severed neck. The head lay near the rubber toe of my basketball shoe, still blinking its eyes. Resting on the precise center of my toe was a bead of ruby blood.

Hack dropped the truncated chicken to the ground, where it ran in frenzied circles spraying a pink mist from the lungs and slinging gouts of darker blood until it finally skidded into a three-point landing, flapped once or twice for good measure, and died. Hack noticed that I had reflexively elevated my shoulders to shelter my neck and was still holding them there, gazing at the blood on my toe. Hack raised his own shoulders and grinned. "You ain't squeamish, are you Doc?"

"No," I said. "I guess I just got a little surprised. I've never seen an animal killed before."

"Well, console yourself that this here is Kinnard's very least rooster, the low one on the totem pole. In the great chicken chain of being he weren't much count."

"How can you know that?"

"He was the lowest one in the tree. You've heard of a pecking order. Well, chickens that roost in trees got a shitting order too. They roost in a hierarchy with the main chicken on top. The top chicken don't catch no shit from nobody, but the bottom chicken gets bombarded by all of it that falls. It's the same kind of game you doctors play. You got the chief of medicine in the top of the tree. Then you got some senior residents squatted on a branch just below and lateral to the chief, and below them are the second year residents squawking and jockeying for position on some limbs. Then below that, you got your interns peeping and ruffling their feathers and trying not to look up any more than they got to while they are participating in that great Darwinian axiom that shit happens downhill." Hack pronounced Darwinian, *Dah-wain-yon.*

"There you go." Hack didn't bother to pluck the rooster; he skinned it and slung the entrails down the ridge, saving the gizzard and the liver. "The Chief may tear me up for throwing away those guts, which he'd use to bait his trotline if he weren't so under the weather. He'd make soup from the head, feet, and the skin. He'd of saved the feathers for a mattress and the bones for stock and telling the future. He'd of done something with everything but the cock-a-doodle-do, which he'd of used already to wake up by."

We made some chicken broth for ourselves and for Kinnard, bland because I wouldn't let Hack add salt or bouillon while the poultry rolled and bubbled in yellow water.

Soon after supper, the diuretics began to work. We helped Kinnard to the porch, where he held on to the post that supported the tin roof and urinated over the edge. This would continue for 12 hours. The old man slept sitting up against the "gunny sack" of corn. He'd call us from his dark corner when his bladder was full, and we'd help him up again.

As Kinnard slept, Hack and I sat on the porch swatting "swamp angels" whose numbers diminished after dusk. We talked and watched fireflies, called *lightning bugs,* spangle the darkness with tiny green lights. We broached many subjects, encountering precious few that Hack couldn't or didn't care to comment on. He was as curious as he was well-informed, and I had been with him often enough to be able to understand his drawl, but the specialized vocabulary that sometimes issued from the mouth of this unlikely intellectual still surprised me, teaching me how deeply rooted is the stereotypical correlation between correct speech and intelligence. Once I'd asked him felicitously to what extent he stressed correct spoken English in Grady Junior High. "Not a bit," he told me, "because they ain't a damn one them who's planning on going over to England. They can read English and they can write it. I ain't gone teach them something in the daytime that they'll get their ass whipped for using at night."

"Well, Doc," he asked now, sipping moonshine on the Gatorman's porch, "if the chief could have got aholt of some foxglove, some *Digitalis purpurea*, would it've cured him?"

"It would have helped him, yes. Dioxin has the same basic ingredient as foxglove, if foxglove is called *digitalis*. In fact, the process we are trying to affect now is called digitalization, but Kinnard's problem is one of severity. His heart is physiologically stressed to the extreme, pumping against the high blood pressure. The heart muscle is like the weaves of a basket. Imagine that the basket is woven from rubber bands. It can expand to pump more efficiently when it has a more difficult job to do, but there is a point where the muscle is stretched too tightly. At this point the heart valves, because they are rigid, don't seal properly. They leak, progressively compounding the edema. Kinnard will die of heart failure in a couple of days if we can't reduce the edema."

"You think you can turn him around?"

"I think so, yes. Tomorrow we'll try to convince him to go with us to the hospital."

"Good luck," Hack said.

"You don't think he'll go?"

"I'll bet you a thousand dollars against them toenails he won't go. He don't even leave the swamp to buy supplies. What he has to have he sends his shine runner for."

"Who is that?"

"Don't your code of ethics prevent you from revealing certain confidential information?"

"Yes."

"Well, mine does too."

"Is it you?"

"Hell, no. I wouldn't of let Kinnard get this sick before I did something. Anyway, I don't run shine, not no more, but I will tell you this: My daddy, Elroy Singletree, used to be the one to run shine for Chief Fish, and I ain't one bit ashamed of it."

"Is it commonly known that Kinnard makes whiskey?"

"Sure."

"Then why doesn't Sheriff Bootman do something about it?"

Hack shut up.

The immediate night was electric with peepers, crickets, and cicadas, but the wider night included the whip-poor-wills' whistle, the jug-o-rum of bullfrogs, and the haunting call of owls. I knew better than to be afraid, but I admit that the night sounds awakened some deeply ingrained foreboding, inherited perhaps from ancient ancestors for whom the night sounds were not irrelevant to survival. Once during the night a bobcat screamed, and my body responded with a stereotypically automatic sympathetic response to primordial fear--my testicles drew up, nesting against my abdominal cavity. My bowels prepared to evacuate.

This response was my body's way of preparing for fight or flight.

"That's just a catymount," Hack said, "a bobcat. You ought to hear a panther. A panther will cold-freeze your blood."

Occasionally there was a separate JUG or RUM that was much louder and deeper than the bullfrogs'. Hack said this was an alligator.

"They make right smart fuss when they're fixing to mate, and the bullfrogs do too. It's a matter of territory. The big alligators and the big frogs run the other males from their area with all that fuss. A bull alligator sounds worse than a lion with all his hellfire fuss and bellowing; he's got to map him out some real estate before the girlie-gators will come. Which is, I might as well go ahead and tell you, the reason me and you ain't got no mates. You ain't got no territory, and I ain't run all the males off mine."

"I knew if I sat here long enough, you'd try to feed me some line of horseshit."

"You can call it horseshit if you want to."

"You never did tell me why Bootman doesn't stop Kinnard from making whiskey," I said.

"How'd you like to wake that old Indian up and tell him it ain't right for him to grow his own corn in his own field? Then take some of that corn and wet it down in a croaker sack until it starts to sprout. Tell him when the tails get about an inch long, he can't put them in water and let it set while a yeast he ain't even added ferments the natural sugar. Tell him he can't cook what the lord himself has concocted, catch the steam off of it, and sell it or drink it either one. You want to tell him he can't do that?"

"No."

"Well Bootman don't neither. Besides the Chief makes world class whiskey. The old way, in a small still, without a sugar run, without any shortcuts. He probably makes whiskey the same way your German-Irish granddaddy did. The chief's whiskey is a monument to American history."

Kinnard's whiskey may have been *right toothsome* to Hack, but it tasted like sulfuric acid to me. I lit a candle and took out my notebook. "What's a sugar run?"

"That's when you add sugar to stretch the batch. When the corn sprouts into malt, it changes from starch to natural sugar, which an enzyme breaks down into alcohol and carbon dioxide during fermentation. 'Course the yeast enzyme will break down refined sugar too, but that's rot gut rum to a master craftsman like the chief. He distills only pure corn products, the chief does."

The first glimmer of dawn was backlighting the dark trees, the birds began chirping, and Kinnard got up to urinate. Hack had cut the top out of a plastic jug Kinnard was urinating into so I could measure his rate of elimination. So far he had eliminated fifteen pints of liquid, and his blood pressure was down to 180/100. His lungs sounded much better, and he had stopped wheezing. The swelling in his legs was going down, and his heart rate was 90. He insisted on getting up and walking without help.

"How do you feel after pissing fifteen pints, Chief?" said Hack. "You ought to feel lighter by about fifteen pounds."

"'A pint's a pound the world around,'" I quoted. "Which is, I guess, about the only advantage the English system has over the metric. A pint of water weighs just about one pound."

"Well, I like the English system better," said Hack. "I know how drunk I'll get on a pint of shine, but there ain't no telling what 568 point 26 cubic centimeters would do to me."

"I bet you've drunk twice that amount since last night."

"Well, that don't count, since we was caught up in such engaging and provocative conversation."

Hack got up, broke wind loudly, and went inside to make some coffee.

We left Kinnard's cabin around 10 a.m. As Hack had predicted, the Indian would not go with us. During the night Hack had told me that I could invite him to the hospital but to make sure I did not ask him to go.

"What's the difference?"

"He knows you probably saved his life. He owes you one, and he's obliged to return a favor," said Hack, beating back brambles along the path. "He ain't got a choice if you ask him to go with us, which ain't fair when you take into consideration how much he hates civilization."

"Funny, I never thought of Grady as being civilized."

"To him it is."

I had foreseen this possibility and had brought a three-month supply of

Hydralazine, Digoxin, and Lasix tablets. Kinnard's tablets cost me less than twenty bucks. "If I leave him some medicine, do you think he'll take it?"

"He might. He knows you saved his ass and he knows you didn't have to."

We left the medicine with the instructions that Kinnard take the Lasix and Digoxin at sunrise, to take the Hydralazine at sunrise *and* sunset. To avoid confusion, Hack drew hieroglyphics on the labels with my ballpoint pen. The moon symbol to the left of the sun symbol indicated sunrise, the moon on the right for sunset.

The old Indian waved as we followed the path up the ridge to where Hack had left his truck. When the path veered right, he continued waving blindly in the same direction. The birds were still chirping. I climbed the ridge with a spring in my footsteps, leaving Hack behind. Although I hadn't slept a wink, I felt good. For the first time since I don't know when, I felt really good. I was already thinking about using the life the Gatorman owed me to get him to a hospital for a lens implant to cure his blindness.

Chapter Eighteen
(May 1983)

In the spirit of community service, Flannigan Construction Company didn't contest the legality of Judge Savage's edict that his crew work on my new office to repay their debt to society. However, the men couldn't afford to work long for nothing, so they threw the trailers together quickly, building steps, breezeways, and annexes in record time. The physical construction, except for the masonry, was finished in a few days, and Hack brought a large black sign that the metal shop students at the junior high had fabricated with elaborate wrought iron frame and ornate white lettering:

DOCTOR OTIS STONE, M.D.
INTERNAL MEDICINE

The office equipment, from centrifuge to mosquito clamps, from intubation kits to rectal specula, had to be ordered from a medical supply house since Wright's trust company would not sell me even a Q-tip from Dr. Hogue's office. I found the bank to be cooperative when it came to lending money for office supplies for a medical facility whose visual assets could be seen from the bank president's office window. The same lending institution that was reluctant to finance a used car for me gleefully picked up the tab for a $3,000 examination table and thousands of dollars of other essential equipment, some of which I had no idea how to use.

My first office patient was Senator Richardson, who had absolutely nothing to do with establishing the office or the practice but whom Commissioner Bill Worthy and Miss Ida, who had plenty to do with the office, invited to cut the ceremonial ribbon and christen the signpost. The senator received a green splinter in his eye when he broke a family-sized bottle of ginger ale over the brick colossus (the size of an upended Oldsmobile) that supported the sign and the mailbox. The soft drink, having been shaken up beforehand by Buster Hogue, had exploded when the senator tapped the corner of a brick. Buster figured that agitated ginger ale would behave more authentically like champagne, and it did. The senator insisted upon being photographed as he exited my office, wearing his newly applied eye patch.

Since his cocktail party Karl Wright had contacted me on four different occasions with lucrative offers to work in various offices, hospitals, and clinics, none of which were within commuting range of Shelly. Wright seemed as intent on getting me out of Grady as Ida Worthy and the town council were on keeping me in. I was still uncommitted to a career of practicing medicine in the rural South, but I wasn't willing to tuck tail and abandon Shelly and my patients either. None of Wright's offers, however financially tempting, would allow me to continue Dr. Hogue's commitment to the people of Grady. I knew enough to realize Wright's healthcare-for-profit system neglected the people who needed health care the most, the kind of folks that crowded into my double-wide office every morning, not to mention edematous blind Indians who wandered around in the Swamp of Toa.

Even if I was going to stay on temporarily in Grady, I was going to have to have a receptionist. I'd always been critical of the office receptionists during training back in Miami. They seemed not to know much about their job; they seemed also not to care. Of course, back then I hadn't learned to appreciate the complexity of a receptionist's job, which among other things involved facing thirty to forty patients and their families each day, sick, scared, in pain, frustrated by delay, worried about not being able to pay their bills. Most of my patients were uneducated and poor. Many were illiterate. There being no public transportation in Grady, a patient needing to see a doctor had to beg a ride from a neighbor in a '64 Ford with an odometer that registered 50,000 miles the third time around. One of my patients saddled a mule and rode in for his appointment. Several drove tractors.

I needed a receptionist who could keep an even flow of patients, but one who could also keep her finger on the pulse of my fatigue, reducing the surge of patients on mornings after I'd been up all night, opening the valve when I was fresh and humming. I needed somebody who could tell when an emergency was really an emergency and a person who could treat everybody who came in, no matter how rich or how poor, with compassion and respect--a receptionist who could read my mind, sound my moods, fathom my fatigue, and gauge my despair. I needed Earlene May Culpepper -- Early May for short -- although it took me a while to realize it.

I knew that an incompetent receptionist in Grady, where people tend to suffer silently and regard sickness as a private matter, could kill more folks than I could save. I didn't need some bimbo who wanted off early some spring afternoon telling a farmer to come back next week if his chest continued to hurt. I needed somebody who realized farmers don't go to the doctor in April unless they're dying.

There were, of course, no trained, experienced medical receptionists in Grady County. Hogue never had a receptionist; he used a meat-market approach. If you got sick, you came in and took a number. First come, first serve, and it was up to you to remember to show up every three months to have your blood pressure checked. This method was cheap and time efficient for the doctor, but compliance was lousy and patients didn't get consistent health maintenance. They didn't get annual pap smears, mammograms, or colon cancer screening.

I needed a different records system than Hogue's too. Dr. Hogue had kept thirty years of medical records on index cards and in his massive brain, which was even now turning to dust in the grave. A typical card would be coded something like "UTI A 4 10 30," which, I learned, meant the patient had a urinary tract infection, that 500 mg of Ampicillin had been prescribed four-times-a-day for 10 days. Implied in the shorthand was the doctor's establishment of the chief complaint, that he had asked pertinent questions, done a proper physical exam, and tested the urine. The 30 after the 10 meant the $30 bill had been paid. On the other hand, the 30 coming before the 10 would mean that the amount was due. The system was brilliant in its efficiency, and it had served Hogue well enough in the days before malpractice suits became popular, but when the Benton boy sued Hogue for amputating his leg, Willetts, Trafford's attorney, took one look at Hogue's index cards and advised him to settle out of court.

I was in the ER when the seventeen-year-old Benton was brought in with a severed femoral artery. I knew Hogue had saved the kid's life, but Hogue had no record to document the need to amputate. The roads to the malpractice courts are paved with good undocumented intentions. I'd learned in Miami that the doctor's first and only defense is his medical records. I was determined to have the best system. Even if I was going to turn it over to my replacement, I was going to set my first office up right.

Early May's telephone voice made Scarlet O'Hara sound like a Brooklyn fishwife. An ebullient divorcee in her forties, she popped gum, dripped costume jewelry, and radiated energy and love wherever she bounced in brightly flowered dresses. I cringed when she answered the telephone: "The sun's a-shining... Jesus loves you!... What ails you, sugar!...Well, I declare!"

But Miss Ida had sent Early May over after I'd interviewed a myriad of politicians' nieces and cousins, upwardly mobile hospital staff, and anxious young women looking for a start in the "health care industry." I wasn't about to send away anybody Miss Ida recommended without giving her a thorough chance.

I soon abandoned attempts to get Early May to say: "You have reached the office of Dr. Otis Stone. How may I help you?"

"That's the way they answer over at Hook's Funeral Home," she protested. She was right. By the time she prefaced my greeting with "Jesus loves you," it did sound like she was selling final services, cheerfully of course. She summed it up: "It don't sound *right*. It don't sound like you give a whispering shit if they get well or not."

I decided, wisely it turned out, to leave her alone, and after three months I didn't care if she whistled Dixie over the telephone. She was wonderful. She could determine my degree of exhaustion better than I could, and when I was far behind schedule, she'd make the patients feel like they'd just got there. She cut up, flirted, sympathized, and "chewed the fat." If Early May's manic voice shattered waiting room serenity, it also dispelled anxiety and temerity among the patients. Concerned by some hellish commotion or other in the outer office, I'd poke my head through the door of the waiting room and find patients grinning widely and Early May hovering over one of them like a bright balloon. She was more than a receptionist; she was morale officer, ambience, cheer. No amount of crabbiness or ill temper from me or my patients could infect or dim her brightness. She made me a far better doctor than I was capable of being alone.

In fact she was too good. She got everyone in who needed to be seen, but Grady needed about eight doctors, not one. Between Early May's open door policy and Miss Ida's beating the bushes to bring in patients--with Shelly and the other EMTs funneling trauma in--I started hospital rounds at 6 a.m., worked the office from eight to eight, then left for the hospital, where I saw patients until ten or eleven at night. I was being butchered, chewed up, and spit back out. It was only a matter of time before I was digested and eliminated too. I had a recurring dream of being at Panama City Beach, Florida, and getting buried by one of those waves that swallow California surfers--a Banzai Pipeline. I'm relaxed and swimming in cool Gulf waters when the monster wave roars over and pushes me under tons of water. I struggle to reach the surface, but in a panic, I realize that in the foam and turbulence I'm not even sure I'm swimming *up*. I wake up in a cold sweat, gasping for breath, usually to the ringing of the phone.

Once the sick and dying got past Early May, they had to be prepped by the nursing department. That's how I remembered the private clinics operating in Miami. My problem was that there were only five RNs in Grady, and they already belonged to the hospital or the health department. The nearest nursing school was in Flint, twenty-five miles away. I had to rely on Shelly and her EMTs to be my "nurses" when they weren't hauling the sick and injured. They were experienced in acute crisis management, but they knew nothing about sterilizing instruments, giving immunizations, prepping women for pap smears, or about quality assurance or problem-oriented medical records keeping.

I quickly realized why the fancy clinic doctors in Miami were so professional and efficient. They paid out big bucks for good nurses.

Of course, I had to establish policies and procedures for everything from giving enemas for sigmoidoscopy to "hostile intruder protocol" for abusive or drunk patients. Shelly thought that I was overdoing it, that I was being anal compulsive and trying to get an A in office management, a nerd. She was probably right, but I'd been trained by perfectionists, and I wanted to maintain their standards. I guess I wanted my chief of medicine to slap me on the back if he ever visited Grady--fat chance. Unless he took up cockfights or frog gigging.

"You can't afford the luxury of perfection," Shelly reminded me. "The perfectionists you are trying to emulate had one quarter the patients and five times the staff. They had Ph. D.'s in medical management and masters degree nurses running the clinics." She was right about that too. Andy Anderson, the hospital administrator at Trafford, offered to help out some, but usually I was too proud even to accept that charity.

After seeing the patients, I had to document what I did. Index cards weren't good enough. I had to have the very best record system available. I dictated every note into a tape recorder. This necessitated finding and hiring and retraining a medical transcriptionist. There were two language barriers to overcome since I spoke *Yankee Medicalese*. After running off two semi-competent secretaries sent over by Miss Ida, I finally realized I would have to accept Digoxin being spelled *Deg-sox-on* until I could train Denise, a young black woman who desperately needed the job to support her disabled mother, four brothers, and two sisters. Denise would cry and beg me not to fire her as I had done the others. Shelly told me she would "cut me off" sexually if I fired Denise, and Early May said she'd stop praying for my immortal soul. Threatened thus in body and spirit, I continued with Denise, who was a willing student, despite her deficient language skills.

But my billing and accounting system was the Achilles heel of a medical office that was already crippled at birth. At least I'd *observed* nurses, receptionists, and medical records technicians during my training. But I'd never seen a patient's bill during my four years at Stanford or my three years of residency training in Miami. I never took a business or accounting course in college, and the nearest I came to business was Introductory Typing when I was a freshman in high school. My professors at medical school and in Miami probably didn't know anything about billing either. They were part of a complex incentive-based reimbursement structure that was managed at the private clinic by Ph.D. medical managers. I was taught to look contemptuously down upon the LMD (the local medical doctor) who was trying to be a businessman and didn't have time to keep up with the latest articles in the *New England Journal*. I'd been taught pure medicine, not practical. I'd bought an accounting system that Early May didn't understand, and my private practice had been "in business" for three months before I realized I had no record of the money collected, the money that needed to be collected, the bills that had been paid, or even who I owed. A visit from a dapper IRS agent convinced me to let Trafford Memorial administrator Andy Anderson take over my business records before the Feds sent me to prison. Well, I had an office. Now what?

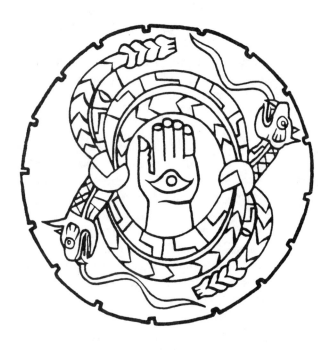

Snake-eye disk illustration

Chapter Nineteen

A mysterious gift about the size of a small pizza appeared on my office steps June 1st in a Wal-Mart bag. It was there when I arrived. When Early May Culpepper came in, I asked her if she knew anything about the reddish stone disk, which was decorated with two rattlesnakes knotted into a circle. Inside the circle was an open hand with an eye in the palm.

"Do I know how it got here, or do I know what it is?" she asked.

"Tell me what you know."

"It's Creek Indian."

"What's it for?"

"I don't know that."

"How did it get here?"

"That neither."

"What else do you know?"

"They's a better one down at the public library."

It was noon before I could leave the office. My last patient was an elderly white woman who'd been treating her rheumatism with polk root, burdock, and white whiskey. After she left, I jogged over to the Grady County Public Library, which was located in the abandoned railway station. Trains hadn't connected in Grady since 1948. Tappie Handson, the librarian, met me at the door. She wore a floral dress with a lace collar. "Shhhh," she said. Her smile raised her cheeks, making slits of her eyes.

"What?"

"Shhh."

"Why? There's nobody in here."

"I'm in here," she whispered.

"Besides you,"

"You're in here, too."

"O.K." I whispered.

"Now, how can I help you?"

"I'd like to see the Native American exhibit."

"What? Speak a little louder, I can't hear you."

"The Indian exhibit," I said, exaggerating my enunciation.

"Follow me," she whispered, walking two steps past me and stopping immediately. "Here you are," she said, gesturing to glass cases that took up a full quarter of the room. "The Native American exhibit is the pride of GPL's holdings, but why are we whispering? As you yourself pointed out, we're the only ones in here."

I smiled, trying to be a good sport. Why was it that everywhere I went somebody was waiting with some kind of practical joke? Unless Shelly was right and it was open season on anybody from anywhere north of Atlanta. Shelly said people teased me because they liked me. She said I was a curiosity, adding that most Yankees who come south are viewed as rude or condescending-- missionaries who come down here to help these poor dumb Southerners and teach them how to "tulk."

I knew Tappie had gone to high school with Shelly, that she had gotten her masters of librarianship at Emory, returning to Grady to care for her mother. "High's yo mamma'n'em?" I said.

"Rat fine. Thankee, Yankee," she said. Her eyes twinkled.

"Do you have anything like this?" I asked, removing my disk from the bag.

Tappie quit cutting up and studied the disk. "We have something similar, yes, but ours is more finely detailed." She led me to another case a few yards away where the refined twin to my rattlesnake disk rested on velour. It was an impressive object of art, slightly concave with carefully incised details on a reddish stone disc, notched at regular intervals around the edge.

"Where did this come from?" I asked.

"Its on loan from Mr. Robert McCormick Jones and Toa Plantation. How Mr. Jones came by it is a story shrouded in mystery, but he claims it was an anonymous gift." Tappie raised her eyebrows conspiratorially. "And I have a question for *you*."

"Shoot."

"Is there anything about the disk of special medical intrigue?"

"Not that I know of, why?" I waited for another leg-pulling.

"Because Dr. Country Trulane, the Flint ophthalmologist, is livid to get his hands on this one. He regularly comes in to drool. Rumor has it he escalates his offer to buy it from Jones in $1000 increments. Of course, Mr. Mack laughs at him. If there's anybody in the world who can't be tempted by money, it's Mr. Mack Jones." Tappie rested her elbow on the display case. "I surmised that Dr. Trulane had a mascot interest because of the eye, and of course the entwined snakes, which suggest the caduceus." Tappie walked briskly to the circulation desk and returned with a key. She unlocked the case and slid back the glass door.

"The what?"

"The caduceus of Hermes, you know, Mercury." She made serpentine gestures in the air and flicked out her tongue. "The staff of Aesculapius, entwined serpents, the symbol of medicine. Don't doctors study liberal arts?"

"Oh, *that* caduceus!" I said. "Listen, tell me about the disk. What does it mean? What did Indians do with it?"

Tappie smiled widely and tilted her head. "Now you are, as we say in the South, barking up the wrong tree. I know next to nothing about Native American artifacts."

"Who does? Besides Dr. A. Hamilton Trulane?"

"A local good ole boy and bucolic intellectual, Hackamore Singletree. Do you know him? Most of this collection belongs to him, except for the snake-eye disk."

"Sure, why did I have to ask?"

"I don't expect if he'll talk to you about the disk. He wouldn't talk to Dr. Trulane."

"Why not?"

"I don't know. Hackamore doesn't have much use for Dr. Trulane. He may not have a reason, or it may be because Dr. Trulane's mother was a Wright. There seems to be bad blood between Hackamore and the Wright family tree, although he was a serious suitor of Beulah Wright before she married Lee Bob Parker. Hack has suffered serious infatuations with more than one Grady belle, though."

"Trulane is from Grady?" I asked, amazed. "The debonair ophthalmologist with the cultured European accent?"

Tappie lifted the disk carefully from the case and placed it on the reference table where the *Readers' Guide to Periodical Literature* was bound in green and lined up by years. "Sure. Country's mother died very young. His daddy was a rural doctor in Graves, a very small town located, as we say, down the road a piece. He died when Hamilton was about sixteen, and Uncle Karl brought Country home to his baronial estate between Grady and Flint. The other kids nicknamed Hamilton Trulane *Country* because Graves was a whistle stop compared to Grady even. "If you drive a buckboard through Graves and sneeze," Tappie said, "you'll miss it entirely."

I learned from Tappie that Karl Wright owned property in Flint and he established residency there so Country and his children could attend Flint schools. She told me that Country was all state in football and basketball in high school and that he would have been valedictorian had he not lost credit in the transfer. He graduated Phi Beta Kappa from the University of Georgia, went to Emory Medical School. Tappie was quite an authority on Country Trulane. And others, it turned out. Like Shelly and Hack Singletree. Southern librarians, she reminded me, specialized in genealogy and gossip.

"After Emory," Tappie continued, "Uncle Karl sent Country to England to study ophthalmology at Oxford, where he took a degree and an imperial bride, much to the disappointment of debutantes in the tri-county area. Country was a flower of Southern manhood. But I'm transcending my role from librarian into that of gossip. I've said enough about subjects I know nothing about, including some of the atypical wildlife of the area, namely Hackamore Singletree."

"I just can't picture Hack Singletree as a ladies' man."

"He never was a *ladies'* man; he just liked women. Still does, I'm told. "

"Did he come around courtin' you?"

"He came around once or twice," she sang. "Yes, he did, with sword and a pistol. "

"How about Shelly Farmer?"

Tappie smiled coyly. "Hackamore is twenty years older than Shelly."

"Shelly is your age, and you were involved with Hack."

"You can ask Shelly about Hackamore, if you aren't afraid of violence." Tappie curved her fingers into claws, threatening me facetiously.

"Why does she hate Hack?" I said, thinking I might as well ask Tappie, since neither Shelly nor Hack had ever been willing to give me a believable answer.

"A lot of Grady girls had crushes on Hackamore Singletree. A beauty and beast motif. Hack was the wildest thing in the county, perhaps the brightest, except for Country Trulane, who was a prince out of our star. Shelly and I were friendly rivals for Hack's attentions about the time we went off to college. Call it father fixation or filial rebellion," she smiled, "but in those days if you wanted to make your parents--excuse the expression--shit and fall back in it, you went out with Hack Singletree. Shelly and I both had adolescent visions of reforming Hack, until we went off to college and realized in the light of academic example just how utterly incorrigible he was. Anybody marrying Hack was going to spend a life fraught with coon dogs, cock fights, and moonshine whiskey, sharing a rickety house with a senile old man and a junkyard for a rear exposure." Tappie spread her arms, smiling. "Then, of course, there was the problem of Beulah. There will always be Beulah."

"Shelly was thinking about marrying Hack?" I felt my jaw drop open.

"Before she went to college, she talked about it, yes, but at UNC she began to realize she and Hack weren't a perfect match, and after her parents died she hated herself for getting mixed up with him in the first place. Hack, in his rough sweet way, wouldn't leave Shelly alone. He mistook her anger for grief and absorbed her abuse. This infuriated Shelly, who thought Hack's dumb male pride kept him from realizing she didn't want him around, but I think Shelly was really more frightened than angry. She was afraid she'd never be able to sort out her feelings and distribute them appropriately between Hackamore and her dead father.

"Girls marry their fathers?" I asked Tappie.

"Unless their fathers die first."

The real irony, according to Tappie, was that Hack wasn't much hurt by Shelly's rejection. He could never understand her interest in him in the first place. It seemed perfectly natural that she come to her senses and dump him.

"Well, there's nothing I'd like better than to stand here all day whispering and chewing the fat," I said, "but I better get back to the office."

"Tell Shelly I said hello," she said. "And Hack."

———————

Country Trulane was waiting for me at my office when I returned from my lunch hour at the library. He wanted to see my rattlesnake disk. When I handed it to him, he seemed humbled and awed. He actually licked his lips. He turned the stone reverently in his hands. "You *know* where it came from," he insisted.

"But I don't, Dr. Trulane. Honest I don't."

"It was just here? I mean, leaning up against your office door?"

"In a plastic bag."

"Where was the bag from?"

"It was a Wal-Mart bag."

"Grady doesn't have a Wal-Mart. The closest one's in Flint."

"That's right," I smiled.

"Listen, you've simply got to sell it to me. I'll pay you whatever you want. I'll give you $5000 right now."

"Dr. Trulane, look. I can't sell it to anybody, at any price, before I know where it came from. I'm not even sure it was intended for me."

"Maybe whoever left it mistook your office for mine," he smiled. "They probably intended it for *me*."

"Your office is in Flint, isn't it?"

"They just took a wrong turn. Seriously, Dr. Stone, I understand your not wanting to sell the disk until you fathom the dark mystery of its origin, but promise me you won't sell it to anyone else without giving me first chance. I'll put up some earnest money for an option."

"I promise," I told him. "We don't need to seal the bargain in money or blood. If I sell it, I'll give you first refusal."

"I don't want you to *give* it away either. "

"No dice. I can't promise not to give a gift, but I doubt I will."

"Fair enough, I guess." Trulane wiped his palms with a silk handkerchief. "Maybe you'll give it to *me*, but as soon as you find out where it came from, let me know."

"That sounds reasonable," I said, "but how did you find out so quickly that I had the disk?"

"I have my sources," said Country Trulane, "and my secrets." His secret was that he had plans to take over Trafford hospital and convert it to an eye surgery center. His first cousin Beulah, who sat on the hospital board, was his major informant of the goings on around Grady. She was also, without my knowledge

97

of the plot, doing her dead level best to pilot Trafford on fiscal rocks to facilitate a Wright takeover. It turned out, however, that Country Trulane found out about my snake-eye disk from Early May Culpepper. Country Trulane, far more than Hack Singletree, was Grady's ladies' man.

Chapter Twenty

Hack turned the snake-eye disk over in his hands and set it down on a table in his study. He produced a pair of wire-rimmed spectacles and put them on his nose, hooking the thin stems around his oversized ears. He pulled a large book from a crowded shelf, leafing through it until he found photographs of Indian artifacts found around Moundsville, Alabama. One page was devoted to rattlesnake disks. One of them, except for the fact that it was more exquisite in detail, was almost exactly like my disk in subject and proportion. I read the description of the Moundsville disk while Hack walked across the room to a wooden footlocker. He returned with an object wrapped in chamois, which he set down and carefully unfolded, revealing another disk that seemed identical to the one in the library and to the one in the book. Hack's disk was at least as accomplished in craftsmanship as the Moundsville carvings. The scales and the rattles of the serpents were intricately depicted, and the human eye, etched into the palm of the open hand, was as carefully and artfully conceived as the textbook artifact.

"There ain't supposed to be none of these snake-eye disks on the east side of the Chatahoochee, according to the book," Hack said.

"Where did you get that disk?"

"It's Daddy's."

"Where did it come from?"

"He don't remember. I found it after Mama died and I was sorting out her stuff. I sent it up to the Smithsonian and had it looked at," he said. "It seems by the patina, or lack of it, to be modern, but it's carved with flint tools."

"How can you tell that?"

He handed me a loupe. "Metal tools, files, make angular grooves. You can see it clearer with a microscope. I went to Moundsville. The carvings are near about identical. The only difference is the three that have turned up around here are ironstone. Sandstone's what one Moundsville disk's made of. The other Moundsville disks are slate."

"What do you think it means?"

"Well, we can bullshit about *that* all you want," he said. "Snakes, because they can shed their skin and renew themselves, have been associated with medicine, immortality, resurrection, and magic since ancient times. They're the princes of the underworld, which is where all of Mother Nature's stores come from. Some scholars think Jewish circumcision dates back to snake worship in the Old Stone Age. The snake gains immortality by sacrificing sloughed off skin, so man was saved by sacrificing a pinch of foreskin. Had enough?"

"Just about," I smiled. I could tell he'd been drinking. He was more grandiloquent under the influence. That and he smelled like a pickled peach. "You can go on a little longer if you'll show a little progress at getting to the point."

"Despite all the bad press the serpent got in the garden of Eden, the Nassenes worshiped Christ as a serpent and celebrated communion by having a snake crawl among the loaves to transform them into the Eucharist."

"What? Early Christian snake-handlers?"

Hack sat down and leaned back in his chair, propping his brogans on the table. "The worshipers passed the snake around kissing it on the mouth. Anyway, the snake's big medicine, and the *bellboy*, as the rattlesnake is affectionately called around here, is the boss snake of the new world, playing big in all Native American hoodoo from the southern U.S. of A. to the Aztecs and Mayas of Mexico and Central America." Hack removed his spectacles.

"These here snakes are tied together into the endless circle, which I reckon represents infinite renewal, some kind of everlasting life, or reincarnation. The hand, I'd guess, is a benedictive guide into the spirit world. A extra eye that ain't in the head represents insight into the inner-self or the hereafter. I'd guess the disk is a ceremonial object for burial. The Moundsville pallets came from burial mounds."

"That's pretty good." I leaned over the two disks and had another look. Each was strangely beautiful in its own way. Each was strangely beautiful in the *same* way too.

"Like I said, I can shovel you a load of horseshit about it like everybody else. But the truth is, don't nobody know."

"Well, since we are involved in idle conjecture, where did mine come from?"

"You ought to be able to figure that one out, Sherlock. What do the three people who got disks have in common? Or who?"

"You mean me, Jones, and your dad, Elroy Singletree?"

"Uh, huh."

"Nothing."

"Yes, you do." He raised a blunt forefinger. "You've all either befriended or offered some service to Potter Fish Kinnard. Jones saved his land, you saved his life, and I don't know what Daddy done, but I do know they're friends, which is somewhere the other side of usual since the chief don't wake up ever morning wanting to make no new buddies."

"Still, he seemed friendly enough. He didn't try to kill us like everybody seemed to think he would," I smiled.

"He was sober and sick. You said yourself he was on his death bed. Dying softens folks up."

"You think Potter Fish Kinnard found those disks along the Capachequi mounds in the Toa?"

"That or he carved them, which would explain why the latest one is sort of rough, him being blind and all." Hack winked.

"In other words, these might be fakes."

"Naw, they ain't fakes."

"Modern, then."

"They ain't modern either, except in the sense that they was carved by a Indian that ain't gone to the happy hunting ground yet. That disk in the book is only five to eight hundred years old. The eye/serpent motif is a archetypal symbol that spans a whole bunch of cultures and goes back thousands of years. If the Chief's making those disks, he's moved by the same spirit that inspired the Moundsville artists. Remember, religious art don't strive for originality. Kinnard's disk is like the Moundsville Disk because the ritual of carving it was passed down authentically to Kinnard. I can guarantee you Kinnard ain't never seen the disk you're looking at from Moundsville, Alabama."

"What's it worth?"

Hack looked like I'd slapped him with a mackerel. "You ain't thinking about selling it?"

"Somebody offered me $5000 today."

"Was it Country Trulane? If it was, he'll go higher than that."

"He made me promise to give him first refusal if I decided to sell. How'd you know it was Trulane?"

"Lucky guess. I don't think you're supposed to sell one of them things a-tall, but I *know* you ain't suppose to sell one of them things to Country Trulane."

Hack picked up a flint projectile point and turned it over. "Look at the back of your hand, Doc. Can you see the eyes in the middle knuckles of your fingers?"

"Uh, sort of." Actually the oval configuration of wrinkles resembled Hack's eyes more than mine, but yes, I could imagine how a primitive mind could find symbolic eyes in his hand.   "What are you saying?" I asked him.

"Nothing," Hack said. "But listen, Doc. You sell that thing, I'm pretty sure you'll screw up the hocus pocus. And I don't think you want to do that. Here, put your hand over the hand on the disk."

At the probable risk of being played the fool, I did it.

"Now line your fingers up with the fingers on the stone and close your eyes."

I did it, feeling very foolish until--maybe it was my imagination--the stone's coolness seemed to rise through my palm, up my wrist, and into my arm. Then there began an almost imperceptible vibration, like an inaudible hum that spread into the right quadrant of my chest, flooding it with warmth. I snatched my hand away.

"Feel anything?" Hack grinned.

"No," I lied.

"Well, that's too bad." He winked a puffy eye. "I'd hoped a big medicine man like you might feel some big medicine. Sometimes I can do that and I'll think I feel some juice and some heat like I just touched a live wire or a pretty gal. But it might be my fancy or the moonshine whiskey I've generally drunk by the time I pull the disk out and start fooling with it in the first place."

"I won't sell it," I promised.

Chapter Twenty-One

S assafras, I'd read, was a diuretic. When I asked Hack about it, he grinned, "Yeah, and it makes you piss a lot too." He walked to an area not fifty yards away and returned with several thin-stemmed shrubs with soft green leaves and pink taproots. After he'd shown me the leaves and stem, and I had pocketed a leaf to copy for my notebook, he broke off the roots. "Boil these up in water and make you some tea," he said, holding the roots under my nose. "They're more potent in winter when the sap's down."

"Smells like rootbeer." I said, wiping grains of sand from the tip of my nose. "Is this as large as they get? Somehow I thought sassafras was a larger plant."

"Yeah Doc, they get bigger than that," he said, pointing to a ninety-foot tree, "but I can't pull that one up."

Later Shelly and I shared a cup of sassafras tea at my kitchen table. She became wistful, recalling her childhood. "I haven't had sassy tea since I was little," she said, entering a nostalgia that included cane grindings, hog killings, and quiltings. As I listened, I was painfully reminded of her convoluted and inextricable ties to this land and its people, to time-honored traditions on the eve of their extinction. I knew I'd never be Southern, and I knew Shelly would never leave the South.

We moved to my front porch and watched the breezes of an approaching early summer storm blow the lake silver and gray. We smelled the ozone and watched cauliflower thunderheads rise beyond the pasture splotched with shadows of dark green. The east wind blew up the underside of the leaves until neon green lightning licked down through towering cumulus clouds.

The change of weather made me pensive and reminiscent, and I spoke of grand cities, of art museums and parks and symphonies and opera and grand cocktail parties and ethnic diversity, cultural richness, and exotic foods. I longed for the tinkle of fine crystal. I was homesick for family and friends, especially my sister Nancy and her husband Jim Maloy, my med school roommate and best friend. But my talk was overpowered by the symphonic onslaught of bullfrogs, peepers, and cicadas, punctuated by the kettledrum and bass of the approaching storm, accompanied by the glissando and tremolo of mosquitoes and mumbling blueflies activated by the lull in atmospheric pressure. When the first big drops fell against the roof, our excitement settled and we held hands, content to listen as the heavier rain assaulted the tin roof. Some of the comfort rain brings is an exemption from duties. Not much can be accomplished during a storm, and absolutely nothing can be done about it.

"I'll bet the cave men made virtually all cave babies in the rain," I told Shelly.

"Cave *women* made the cave babies," she corrected, "but you're probably right about the rain. There's something about the sound of it that makes you feel, uh, procreative."

Philosophic musings gradually turned from anthropological speculation to happy and shameless lust. I suggested we put Shelly's grandmother's quilt to licentious application. Shelly led me by the fingertips to the brass bed we'd bought at a flea market and covered with Granny's homecrafted finery. Above the bedposts, framed and hanging on the wall, was a hand stitched message Shelly had sewn during the long hours between emergencies: REMEMBER ME? I'M THE ONE YOU SLEPT WITH LAST NIGHT!

She undressed and lay on her side against the patchwork quilt. Her tawny, close-cropped head propped on her elbow, her hip raised by that wonderful anatomical distinction particular to post-pubescent daughters of Eve--the wide pelvic girdle. I marveled as the dappled light from the rain-spattered window projected raindrops upon the incandescent flesh of this woman I was so helplessly and breathlessly beginning to love. I was content to lie there watching her for many long moments.

"Let's play doctor," she smiled. Tucked in, we listened to the driving hiss of rain as the muted twilight darkened into night. I knew that wherever Shelly was, there was my home.

Chapter Twenty-Two

That July when her great granddaughter Cyrilla brought Miss Ethel Hargrove to me with a pulmonary embolism, her fourth episode in the last five years, Miss Ethel bore her pleuritic pain with such dignity that Nurse Holt and I didn't recognize at first the severity of her condition. "Big Mamma cain catch her breath and she sick to her stomach," Cyrilla reported. "She say she gone die."

The old woman was of the natural coloring other blacks called *redbone*, honey-complected with the faintly reddish tint of heart pine. Of course, that midnight in the emergency room, she was gray as salt water taffy.

A wide-framed and angular woman, she carried herself into the hospital with the same monumental presence she had when I first saw her in Dr. Hogue's office months before his death. Her large kind hands upon her walker, she was gasping deeply for breath.

"So you're ninety-nine," I said, sitting her down. "You don't look a day over ninety-six."

Miss Ethel smiled above her pain, and I could tell by that smile that she was a woman accustomed to status and affection.

"Does it hurt you very much, ma'am?"

"Yes, Doctor, it surely do." Her face glowed with perspiration, and the deep splintered lines from her eyes deepened with discomfort, but her quiet grace gave me the uncanny feeling that she was somehow partially immune to the agony of us common mortals, as though she had weathered and endured to some higher plateau where anguish and death were not strangers or enemies to her. She seemed utterly without fear, although I knew she must be having a fright response, the panicky feeling of impending and unavoidable doom that accompanies a pulmonary embolism.

"How many children do you have?" I asked, realizing that her children could have died long ago of old age.

"I raised . . . nineteen," she smiled. "My husband had . . . nine children when we married . . . . Him and me found ten."

"Found?"

"Begat," translated Margaret Holt.

"How many grandchildren?" I asked.

Miss Ethel smiled.

"She don't know," snapped Nurse Holt. "She need to get her some oxygen and some medicine for her pain and her dyspnea!"

"What kind of medications are you taking?" I pretended to ignore Margaret Holt.

"Here they," said Cyrilla, handing me a bottle of ordinary aspirin and a brown bottle of homemade beige pills that looked to have been rolled in the palm of Big Mamma's hands.

"What are these? Who told her to take this?"

"She tell herself what she take."

"Anything else?"

"She take three cups of rosemary and sage tea," said Cyrilla. "She have one glass of garlic water in the morning. She have a ginkgo tree in her yard. She chew up some leaves in the evening to keep her mine fit."

"Is your mind fit, Miss Ethel?"

"Sho it is," the old woman gasped. "When the elephants cain't recollect something, they comes to see me."

I did an arterial blood gas, inserting a syringe into a radial artery in her wrist. The blood pushed up the plunger, showing that the needle was into an artery, but the blood wasn't bright red arterial blood. It was purplish, indicating a physiologic shunt--her blood was passing through her lungs without getting oxygenated.

Nurse Holt gently inserted oxygen tubes into Miss Ethel's nose.

"I know you are experiencing a fright response, feelings of impending doom," I told Miss Ethel, "but that results from the hypoxia. Those feelings will disperse as soon as we can get some oxygen in your blood."

"You think you gone die, but you ain't," Nurse Holt translated loudly.

"I know . . . what the young doctor say," Miss Ethel smiled sadly, "and I thanks him . . . for his kindness . . . and his help."

"She gone die," moaned Cyrilla, her cheeks slick with tears. "She *know* she gone die."

"Hush child," said the old woman, "You know I has been . . . a long time . . . on this earth."

The EKG showed atrial fibrillation and M-shaped patterns in the first chest lead of right ventricular strain. I'd suspected a moderate to large embolism. If I'd had a radiologist available, I'd have gotten a lung scan. *If a frog had wings*, Hack's voice mocked me, *he wouldn't skin his ass on a three-point landing.*

"I want to transport you to Putnam Memorial Hospital in Flint," I told Miss Ethel.

She shook her head. "My soul have . . . enough trouble getting home from this place here."

"You'll be better off at Putnam," I insisted, "safer."

She still refused to go. "No suh," she smiled, "Once you get Grady . . . County dirt in your shoes . . . it hard to shake it out."

Well, that's the damn truth, I thought. I've been trying to get Grady dirt out of my shoes since my car blew a water pump on the interstate. This place sucks like a black hole. Nothing, not even light, leaves Grady.

From Margaret Holt I discovered that Dr. Hogue had treated the patient on three occasions for pulmonary embolism and thrombophlebitis. We switched her from tubes to a 100% oxygen re-breather and started an IV Heparin drip, but I wanted to consult at least one experienced specialist to hold my hand on this one. I had no idea what happened to hundred-year-old blood when it was thinned with powerful anticoagulants. At 1:30 a.m. I woke up Dr. Phillip Mendenbalm, Flint oncologist and hematologist, and told him I had a ninety-nine year-old female patient with a clinical suspicion of pulmonary embolism. "Her PO 2 is 46, oxygen saturation is 75 percent," I said.

"Put her on 100% oxygen, start a Heparin drip, and get her over to Putnam right away," ordered Dr. Mendenbalm.

"I've started the oxygen and heparin, but she won't go. She's afraid her soul will take the wrong exit off the perimeter road. She's lived nearly a century without leaving Grady County, and she's seen enough on T.V. to convince her to stay put and appreciate a good thing."

"You've told her, of course, that Flint is the 'Good Life City' and that Dr. Phillip Mendenbalm is the foremost hematologist and faith healer on the planet."

"Of course I've told her all that, but she still won't go."

Mendenbalm paused. "Well, after you get her through the crisis, you'll have to convert her to Coumadin."

While I was at it, up and about after the witching hour, rousing my colleagues with 2 a.m. wake-up calls, I figured I might as well endear myself to Dr. Jeffery Roberts, a chain-smoking thoracic surgeon who wrote poetry and drove motorcycles.

"Yeah," he said, clearing his throat with a sound like a restaurant size coffee percolator, "which son-of-a-bitch is this?"

"This is Dr. Otis Stone at Trafford in Grady. I'm sorry to have to wake you up, but I've got a large pulmonary embolism I need to consult with you about."

"Oh, you didn't wake me up," growled Roberts. "I was watching the light squiggles on the back of my eyelids. After that I was going to count the raisins in the goddamn cereal." There was a long pause, then a coughing fit. Then another long pause while Roberts, presumably, stuffed his own lungs back down his throat.

"Listen Dr. Otis Stone, transport your patient over to Putnam. We'll need lung scan and pulmonary artiogram. Then we'll fish the clot or dissolve it with Streptokinase."

"Dr. Roberts, the patient is a ninety-nine-year-old black female who refuses to be transported."

"Whoa son," said Roberts. "Ninety-nine! Christ, consult with *her*, not me. I'm damn near dead at forty. Listen, any kind of surgical procedure at her age is very risky. If she was maybe a half century younger she might be a candidate for an embolectomy." Roberts paused for about the time it takes to fumble a cigarette from a bedside table and light it. "Maybe we could get by with a ligation of the inferior vena cava," he said, "or maybe we could put a Greenfield filter in, but you got a tough choice, cowboy, and you want to go along with her wishes. I guess I'd try IV Digoxin, oxygen, Heparin, and prayer."

"Do I do a long-term anticoagulation?" I asked. "Should I convert her to Coumadin to prevent another clot from forming? Since she's had three, another one might kill her."

"Yeah, get her through the crucial part and ask her again about an operation, but don't push her. The rules change with patients over 98. I mean, make sure she's comfortable. Shit! How many years can you expect to prolong the life of a hundred-year-old woman?"

"Ninety-nine," I corrected.

"Yeah, well keep me posted, and good luck."

"Thanks, and again, I'm sorry about waking you up."

"No sweat, I had to get up anyway to answer the goddamn telephone."

It took three days to stabilize Miss Ethel. Whenever I was at the hospital and found myself with a moment between patients, I couldn't resist the temptation to chat with someone whose life and memory had spanned nearly a century. I recorded this entry in my notebook:

Her father was born "the year after freedom," in 1866. Her mother died when Mrs. Hargrove was 13. Being the eldest daughter, she raised the younger children, for her father refused to distribute his children to relatives as was the custom. Her father was a hard working, hard drinking man who went to school for only five months but who could "read the bible and tend to his bidness." He hunted, fished, trapped, and farmed, raising cotton and corn. "We growed peanuts too," she said, "but folks growed peanuts to feed the hogs. Folks didn't grow peanuts much for eating. Us dried what we wanted to eat on the roof of the house." Her father would not let his children visit "the quarter" nor would he allow young men from the quarter to "come around to court me," cursing and threatening them until they went away. He arranged her marriage to a widower with nine children, whom she was able to survive after a measly couple of decades. When there was a smallpox, malaria, or influenza epidemic, she remembered, "coloreds" were stacked like cordwood and taken to town. The doctor would come outside and see them on the buckboard, but they weren't allowed inside. She recalled treating her brother's recurring knee and elbow pain by applying a flannel cloth soaked in a mixture of kerosene and turpentine. "The heat seemed nearly always to ease off the pain."

The waiting area outside Miss Ethel's room soon became crowded with family and well-wishers--men, women, and children--who kept an around-the-clock vigil. I ordered that her visitors be limited to immediate family. Nearly a hundred people lined up in the hall with flowers, fried chicken, and cake.

"Those peoples *is* her immediate family," said Margaret Holt. "At least those the ones had time to get here from where they stay." It appeared that Miss Ethel's immediate family could fill up the Grady High School gym.

Cyrilla would not leave her great grandmother's side, so we put a cot in Room 47, The Benbow Hutchinson Memorial Intensive Care room, and let her stay. She and Nurse Holt acted as intermediaries, keeping the waiting room congregation informed of Miss Ethel's progress. Men in black suits and vests sat solemnly around while women in flowered hats and dresses arranged food and flowers and governed children. Little girls in pink and white Easter dresses had pigtails plaited so tightly that I doubted they could close their eyes. Little boys ran around in short pants and white shirts, tamed by older sisters who slapped at them and cried "*Be*-have." The group's organization was largely matriarchal, except for the preacher, who periodically led the group in prayers and muted songs.

"Can't we do something about some of this?" I asked Margaret Holt. "This is turning into a circus. What are all these people doing here?"

"They here to honor Miss Ethel when she pass."

"What? Do they think we are giving her some kind of test?"

Nurse Holt marveled at my ignorance. She watched the overhead fan. "To pass mean to die."

"Well, she's not going to die, at least I hope she isn't."

Then it occurred to me that Nurse Holt and the others might know something about Miss Ethel that I didn't. "She isn't going to, uh, pass, is she?"

"If she decide to pass, she will pass," Nurse Holt said gravely. "Miss Ethel always do what she say she gone do."

"Well, please go tell her she's not going to."

"You go tell her. You her doctor."

"Well, you're going with me." I still didn't feel totally comfortable communicating across cultures without a translator present.

When we entered Room 47, Cyrilla was fanning Miss Ethel with a cardboard fan provided by Stokes Funeral Home. It had a picture of a white Jesus in the foreground and Martin Luther King, Jr., behind him in the clouds. Both icons had yellow haloes. I noticed that Cyrilla had planted African violets in the bedpan. "You are not going to, uh, pass," I told Mrs. Hargrove.

"We give you some pills to spread out your blood, Miss Ethel," said Margaret Holt. "You'll make it right on."

"She must be very careful about hurting herself," I told Cyrilla. "The Coumadin will thin her blood. A minor cut could cause severe bleeding."

"You got to watch you don't hurt yourself," said Margaret Holt.

"Big Mamma can stop blood," said Cyrilla compressing her lips and nodding definitively.

"How?" I asked.

"Big Mamma, she can stop the blood with her mind, but if she don't, I puts on spider web and soot."

"Will that work?" I asked Margaret Holt.

"Every time," she said. "The web clot the blood and the soot dry it up and make a scab."

"Very well. Now Nurse Holt, please go out there and tell those people that Ethel Hargrove is not going to die and they can go home."

"*You* go tell them that; you still the doctor, and every one of them peoples speaks English."

I wasn't going to lose another standoff to Margaret Holt. I took her hand firmly and led her by Rev. Peace, whom I snagged, taking them both to a table at the front of the waiting room. I clanked a wooden spoon against a bowl of potato salad until the room quieted and I had the attention of every man, woman, and child. "Nurse Holt, Reverend Peace, and I have an important announcement to make: Miss Ethel Hargrove has decided not to pass at this time. Reverend Peace will lead us in a brief prayer of thanksgiving after which . . . ."

"And one spiritual," Reverend Peace interjected, tilting his head to the side.

". . . and one short spiritual, after which we will file quietly out of the waiting room, down the hall, down the stairs, into the parking lot and into our automobiles, so that we may follow the ambulance procession to the Hargrove home, where we will continue to celebrate Miss Ethel's good health."

Margaret Holt almost smiled. At least, for a flickering moment her perpetual scowl lightened.

"Nurse Holt, after the prayer and the spiritual, will you arrange for Mrs. Hargrove's release from Trafford and summon Miss Farmer and the ambulance to transport her home?" I formally requested, loud enough for all attending to hear.

"Yes, Doctor," Margaret Holt said. I thought I was going to swell up and float off. Margaret Holt had actually spoken respectfully to me in front of other people. I felt better than I had the day I received my M.D. degree. This was really something.

110

Chapter Twenty-Three

The first time I'd seen Wilkin Wright since his father's cocktail party, his brother Marvin brought him comatose into the hospital. Even against the pallor of his complexion, I noticed that Wilkin had a waxy scar the color of crab meat, which began at the bridge of his nose, circumcised its wing, then disappeared into the nostril of the opposite side. Hack's signature, which Hogue had closed with the family physician's un-cosmetic efficiency, was upon him like the mark of Cain. His brother's front incisor plate was falsely framed in gray. I briefly pictured Hack gagging Marvin with his .44 magnum to make Marvin regurgitate narcotics evidence for Rooster Bootman and knocking off Wilkin's nose. When I'd seen the boys stealing tequila from Wright's patio bar, I hadn't gotten a good look at the effects of Hack's handiwork. Now, viewing the scar tissue resulting from his attack, it seemed even more incongruous to Hack's character that he was capable of violent acts against fellow human beings.

Wilkin's deep and rapid breathing, loss of skin turgor, and acetone breath led me to recognize the symptoms of diabetic ketoacidosis, but even before I saw the brothers, Margaret Holt had made the diagnosis. She charged into my office like a linebacker, "Wilkin Wright, history of diabetes, out cold and sucking wind. He got slack skin and a white ring around his mouth; he stink like fruit cocktail. Diabetic ketoacidosis."

"That's pretty good, Mrs. Holt," I said as I examined Wilkin, "pretty damn good."

I rubbed Wright's sternum, then raked his shinbone, getting no response. "Start an 18 gauge angiocath STAT!" I told Nurse Holt. "Hang normal saline and let her rip as fast as she'll go. Then get me an SMA-18, a blood gas, serum acetone, and a CBC. And tell Billy Simmons to get his fat ass out of bed and into the lab. I want serial SMA-6's until this patient is out of ketoacidosis." Billy was Trafford's lab technician.

There was nothing like a good case of diabetic ketoacidosis to get an internist inspired and motivated. This severe derangement of metabolism was once 100% fatal. Even in good hands it still carried a mortality rate of 10%. Here was a case to show my stuff. One of the rare situations where the internist is able to save a life within a couple of hours like his surgical colleagues--to outshine for once the venerable family doctor, Hogue.

I wanted to make sure Nurse Holt appreciated my expertise, so I continued barking orders like I was reciting a chapter out of *The Manual of Medical Therapeutics*: "Give ten units of regular insulin IV, then start a regular insulin drip at ten units per hour. Insert a foley cath, place him on telemetry, and do fingerstick blood sugars q. 1 hour. Get three sets of blood cultures and a urine

C&S; then start Ancef 1 gram q. 8 hrs. After the first liter of saline is in, give another one at 500 cc's an hour, then one at 250 cc's an hour. By that time we should be adding some dextrose and potassium."

To my surprise Billy got me an SMA back within 30 minutes showing a bicarb of 4 and a potassium of 3.6 and a sugar of 856--profound ketoacidosis and a life-threatening deficiency of potassium.

"Stick 40 milliequivalent of K in the liter of saline that's running."

Nurse Holt froze.

"What's the matter?

"You got me giving him something he don't need."

"What do you mean, Mrs. Holt? I could treat DKA in my sleep. Follow the orders I gave you."

"This ain't the way we treat ketoacidosis."

"Who's we?"

"Me and Dr. Hogue don't."

"Well, Dr. Hogue is dead, and this is the way we treat ketoacidosis, you and Dr. *Stone*, and we do it right away, goddamn it."

Margaret Holt, not to be intimidated, crossed her arms, standing solidly in her tracks. I knew what that meant. She'd stand right there until Hooks came down to embalm Wilkin and Karl Wright selected a coffin. I decided to try detente. "Listen Margaret, I know what I'm doing here. I lack experience in a lot of areas, and ordinarily I appreciate your guidance, but on the observation unit where I trained, I treated three or four DKA's a day. After establishing the protocol I'm asking you to follow, I never lost a patient. Can you say *that* for the procedure you and Dr. Hogue followed?"

"No, we never gave no potassium, and this man don't need none."

"That's why you and Hogue probably lost 15-20% of your DKA's," I told her, pointing to the potassium reading on the lab report. "Your patients seemed fine at first, didn't they? Then within 12 hours they died. Acidosis artificially raised the potassium count so that the deficiency went unnoticed, becoming fatal."

I finally convinced Nurse Holt that I knew what I was talking about. My protocol was simply more up-to-date than Hogue's, one of the advantages of studying modern medicine three decades later than Hogue did. Still, I could not free myself from his watchful ghost. The old doctor walked with me and watched over my shoulder. Six months after his death he was still there for every treatment and every procedure. When I seemed to be talking to myself, I was really talking to him, seeking his approval, caring for patients who came with his territory and had belonged to him. Some who still owed him money were remitting to me, causing a bookkeeping fiasco for Early May, who had to separate those fees and forward them to Hogue's widow.

Within twelve hours, Wilkin was alert. His bicarbonate was back to normal; his potassium fell only to 3.2, but he had no arrhythmias because the potassium supplement was started early.

Late that night as I left Wilkin's room, I saw a large man in a Stetson and a safari jacket at the end of the hall. Hack! I called, but the figure dissolved into the stairwell shadows. He sure looked like Hack, but, I guessed, any giant in a cowboy hat and a safari jacket would look like Hack. How many giants were there in Grady who wore cowboy hats? I was too tired to give the coincidence much thought, but as I passed the nurses' station, Margaret Holt stopped me.

"Hack Singletree find you?" she asked.

I paused, turned, and ran to the stairwell, pulling myself by the rail as I vaulted the steps three at a time. A high, loud scream reverberated down the corridors of the second floor.

"Help! Nurse! Help! Noooo!"

Charging down the empty hall into Wilkin's room, I expected to find Hack ripping out Wilkin's IV, but how could he have guessed that without potassium supplementation Wilkin could die. Maybe he overheard me arguing with Margaret Holt about the IV? Knowing Hack, he could have read about potassium in the *New England Journal of Medicine.* But when I bolted through the doorway to Wilkin's room, Hack was not ripping out Wilkin's windpipe or his IV's. He was smiling at Wilkin, grinning like a bulldog and snapping on a pair of latex gloves. I'd never seen a smile that bore such unearthly and murderous glee.

"Hack! Whoa!" I yelled.

The patient's body was locked in a sitting position, his mouth and eyes were wide open, and every fiber of his body registered mortal fear. He grabbed up his sheets and bunched them beneath his chin in a movement that yanked out his IV and exposed his thin, vulnerable feet. "Help!" he screamed again. Hack, who was bent over at the waist, straightened up and turned to face me, his murderous smile melting back into a more typically hayseed, dumbass look. But I would never forget that sinister, prognathic leer. Except for the eyes, the expression was one you would expect to find on the face of a corpse that had just met a hideous death. The eyes radiated pure, living hatred.

I rushed past Hack to the bedside of Wilkin Wright. Finding a vein in the top of Wilkin's hand, I reinserted his IV and buzzed the nurses' station. Then I shoved Hack roughly from the room. "What are you doing?" I demanded. He was easier to push around than I expected, perhaps a little off balance from drinking. More likely he was incapable of reacting physically to a friend.

"Nothing!" His grin became more natural. He ducked his head and raised his arms in mock defense. "Just paying this boy a visit. It's visiting hours, ain't it. He must be delirious, though. He's done got upset and scratched his IV a-loose," he laughed. "I was getting ready to call Nurse Holt to see did the boy need something to calm his young ass down." Hack's *ass* sounded like ice. He smelled like a bucket of rotten pears.

"What are you doing here, Hack? You could go to jail for assault. What in the hell are you thinking about?"

"Preventive health care."

"What?"

"You taught me about that. In the long run, that boy in yonder's going to be better off if he stays out of Grady. I was just reminding him to keep to a more healthful climate."

"Wilkin can't help being here. I put him in the hospital."

"If he'd been hanging around somewhere else when he got sick, he'd gone to another hospital."

"Well, I don't understand what goes through your mind to make an educated man act like a redneck thug."

"Bryan Cheek and Yolanda Cousins." His red-rimmed eyes became serious and dull like a goat's eyes.

"Who's that?"

"Bryan's an eighteen-year-old kid who got strung out on crack cocaine. He shot his parents in bed and slit his sister's throat. Yolanda's a fifteen-year-old chicken head, a girl who performs group fellatio for drugs."

"A chicken head?"

"So called for the jerky movement of her head when she's sucking off her suppliers."

"How is Wilkin responsible?"

"There wasn't no crack cocaine in Grady before this maggot got to dealing it."

"Does Wilkin smoke crack?"

"Naw, he snorts coke, which he affords by supplying crack to street dealers. They hawk it to prostitutes and teenyboppers in Flint. If he was to go ahead on and die, it would be a boon to mankind, but I didn't do nothing but smile at the little cocksucker."

"I saw that smile. You clearly intended to do harm to my patient."

"Now, Doc," Hack said, flashing that same diabolical leer then wiping it off. "Like Shakespeare says, there ain't no art to find the mind's construction in the face. How do you know what I was up to. That smile is my umbrella. I keep it in

114

my hip pocket for a rainy day."

"Haw!" Margaret Holt brushed by us, flashing a don't-mess-with-me look of her own.

I didn't know what to do. Even though I had just seen him counterfeit the horrible expression that made me fear for Wilkin's life, that look alone had now convinced me of what Shelly had been telling me all along, that Hack was potentially dangerous. I felt duty bound to call the sheriff and duty bound not to. Practically speaking, there wasn't any proof that Hack intended to assault Wilkin, certainly not enough to move Rooster to arrest his friend. Then too, of course, Hack was my best friend. I didn't want to put him in jail and be the one to go right back down there and bail him out. I decided to bluff.

"Well, I'm going to tell you right now my first loyalty is to the welfare of my patients. I want your word of honor that you'll leave this hospital and not return as long as Wilkin Wright is a patient here. I know there's a court order forbidding you to knowingly intrude into the whereabouts of Wilkin or Marvin Wright. You've violated that order by coming here today so that you stand now in contempt of court. You know that I can have you arrested."

"You'd of made a good lawyer, Doc, but I'd tell Rooster Bootman I was looking for you. How'd I know where that little shitass was?"

"If you come around here again, I'll tell Beulah Parker you're harassing her little brother."

"Color me gone," Hack grinned, "but there ain't nothing wrong with your patient in yonder . . . ."

"That a little killing won't cure?"

"There you go."

Before I finished my rounds, I passed back by Wilkin's room and found him gone. I went by the nurses' station and asked Mrs. Holt about him.

"He gone," she said. "He called Marvin to come at him."

"He can't be gone. I haven't released him yet."

"He gone," she assured me. "It was Hack released Wilkin. He grinned Wilkin right on out of here."

I was furious. "What?" I shouted. "Hack didn't come back by here, did he?"

"Naw. He grinned him good enough the first time."

"He didn't just grin. He must have threatened him in some way. He must have told him something."

"Hack told Wilkin he thinking about snatching his adenoids out his ass."

That would have done it, I thought. Hack's drunken grin looked like Mr. Hyde with a hangover.

115

Chapter Twenty-Four

My second meeting with Beulah Parker, Lee Bob's seductive wife and Hack's mistress, occurred that August at a Trafford Memorial Hospital Authority meeting under not so pleasant circumstances. As a matter of fact, my decision to send an infected foot to Flint, at a time when Trafford was $300,000 behind in revenues, was not perceived well by the board, who had to call on the county's emergency fund to make payroll. Andy Anderson, the hospital administrator, called me into his office beforehand for the summons.

"You may be the best hotshot to have around when I have my miocardial infarction," he began, "but you'll be the one who'll give me that goddamn coronary, too."

"Don't start about the Marberry girl. I'm not a goddamn pediatrician."

"Otis, she's ten years old. Girls have babies in this damn county when they're ten years old, and she had an infected bone in her foot for Christsake, an infected foot. Do you know what they are doing for her over at Putnam, where you transferred her?"

"Yes, Oxacillin 1.5 grams every four hours."

"That's just fancy penicillin. Why can't we give it to her? Listen, Putnam is going to keep her 42 days at $300 a day, 100% of which is covered by Blue Cross. Your decision to transfer her is going to cost Trafford over $10,000, not to mention pissing off Curtis Marberry, the biggest pecan farmer around here. How do I know he'll be pissed? Because he came into my office this morning pissed. His wife is going to have to stay at the Holiday Inn for six weeks. The way he sees it, you've split up his family and cost him a shitpot full of money for Putnam to administer a medicine he can buy for his hogs over the counter at the veterinarian supply."

My heart went out to Andy Anderson. Trafford was his first hospital, and he'd had nothing but bad luck. Hogue's death and Benbow Hutchinson's changed will had nearly administered a *coup de grace* to a hospital that was floundering in the first place. Before Benbow Hutchinson died, Trafford was hanging on to the hope of his promise of a $4,000,000 legacy. Then a young massage parlor entrepreneur, Denise Carswell from Phoenix City, Alabama, arrived on the scene. Denise married the 88-year-old philanthropist, whom she subjected to insupportable ecstasy, effecting a new will and her benefactor's demise. Denise left town before the funeral.

Andy Anderson had to lay off over 20% of the staff, including the chairman of the Authority's niece. The hospital census was down 50%. If Trafford went under, Anderson would be head of housekeeping in a big hospital for the next ten years before he could move up the chain of command to a managerial position of the magnitude he held now, which wasn't much.

The very last thing in the world I wanted was to participate in destroying Trafford. I was an internist, and an internist was nothing without a hospital. Trafford provided a great community service, no doubt about that, especially for the poor country folks, black and white, who would *lay down and die* before they'd leave the county and their families to be sick in a far away city 20 miles from home. But the Marberry girl rested on the other side of a line I wouldn't cross. I was licensed in the state of Georgia as a physician and surgeon, but I was qualified to practice only adult medicine, and medically speaking the girl with the infected foot was a child who required the services of a pediatrician. I was determined not to go beyond my *comfort level*, although I knew there were plenty of doctors who crossed the line every day for just such practicalities as Anderson and I were discussing now. I'd sworn never to let economics sway my professional judgement, and Chrissy Marberry was just going to have to be a case in point.

"There's to be a meeting of the entire Hospital Authority at one p.m. sharp. Just cancel your patients and get your ass over there, Otis. I've asked Flowers to cover your calls and see the emergencies."

Whatever else the hospital authority meeting meant, after the inquisition I'd have an afternoon off to spend with Shelly--my first real afternoon off since Dr. Hogue's death seven months before. I called her and asked her to swap some time with Buster or another EMT and meet me at Loonie Lake mid-afternoon. She'd get somebody to shuttle her to my house in the ambulance, then I'd catch a ride after the meeting. I was going to have to get a car of some kind.

"What's up?" Shelly said. "Are you going to stamp out all the disease in the county before the 12 o'clock whistle?"

"Emergency meeting of the Authority."

"Uh, oh. Marberry?"

"That's part of it."

"Well, just keep your lower mandible elevated and tell them you're not a pedophile and you don't do windows. I'll fix a nice dinner and we can mess around if your testosterone level hasn't dehydrated into desert dust."

"It's a pediatrician," I said, "that I'm not."

"Then you *are* a pedophile? I wouldn't tell them about that. Everyone is entitled to a little perverse privacy. On second thought tell them *maybe* you'll do the windows. And that you'll do the Marberry girl too, the instant she reaches puberty or gets a zit. Whichever comes first."

"Goodbye," I said. Shelly was dutifully supportive, but she was only slightly more sympathetic than the hospital authority had promised to be. She wasn't inclined to draw too fine a line between ten-year-old girls and twelve-year-old.

She believed when there was a job that needed doing, the first one on the spot should roll up her sleeves and get moving. She didn't believe in investing in a lot of high-tech fiber optics necessary to split hairs. Of course Shelly could afford a Samaritan attitude better than I could. She lived closer to emergency. Do something NOW even if it's wrong. But my predicament with Marberry wasn't a matter of life and death as much as a matter of ethics. That and an acute reluctance on my part to spend the first year of my career in a malpractice suit.

Hack understood Shelly's feelings, although Shelly had--in Tappie's words-- become *acutely intolerant* of Hack since her parents' death, but Hack bore no malice for Shelly. He defended her actions and her attitudes as though out of mutual admiration. "She wants you to fish or cut bait and let somebody else discuss the dynamics of piscatology," Hack had said in an apology of Shelly's hotheaded condemnation of my professional floundering.

"What do you mean?" I'd asked him.

"She's got the idea that you think the best doctors are the ones furtherest removed from somebody sick," he'd answered. "And she's dead right." He pushed his open hands into his hip pockets. Then, turning around, he wiggled his fingers to create the illusion that his ass was twitching uncontrollably, a gesture he used when he wanted to mix levity with constructive criticism.

"Well, I'm not going to discuss the finer points of practicing academic medicine with somebody who goes to the vet for snakebite."

Hack looked back over his shoulders, grinning and wiggling his fingers. If I'm destined to remove marbles from the beshitted assholes of juveniles for the rest of my career, I thought, I'm at least determined to do it in more important academic medical centers than Trafford Memorial. When I expressed this sentiment to Hack, he countered, "City folks got assholes too," he teased. "I hear out in L.A. they got them on both ends."

The hospital authority board room reflected the general state of Trafford. The walls were faded yellow with cracked plaster and peeling paint. The floors were linoleum. From the slowly revolving overhead fans, curls of flypaper studded with houseflies waved in the breeze. The thermostat was turned up to 85 degrees, presumably to emphasize the fiscal dilemma of the hospital, and all ten of the board members seated at the long table sweated and spit gnats, except one-- Beulah, who stared at me so long and intently with long-lashed and hooded eyes that I checked to see if my fly was zipped. This *femme fatale* with luscious cleavage and stiletto fingernails bright as arterial blood was none other than the notorious Beulah Wright Parker. I was seated directly across the table, and I confess that I was more than a little moved by her sexuality. In her mid-forties,

118

she sat in an aura of plush sensuality that transpired from her pores. Her bright lips widened into a slow and easy smile as she reached across the table to renew our acquaintance.

"I'm happy to see you again," she said, squeezing my hand with bejewelled and manicured fingers that suggested velvet over sinews of steel.

The board chairman, Morton Willetts--a thin, gray-haired man with a rodent profile and hound-dog eyes--spoke first. Besides being the authority board chairman and the hospital attorney, he represented Wright, at least to the extent that he handled Wright's interest in Hogue's office. His posture, which would have been a screaming conflict of interest in Washington, was considered business as usual in Grady, where everyone knew there could be no serious conflict of Willetts' interest since Willetts' interest was always clearly his own. The fact that his fingers were in virtually every pie was viewed more as mildly incestuous than contradictory and no more reproachable than marrying a first or second cousin.

"Dr. Stone," he said, "all of us appreciate your good, diligent work here in the county. We know that this is not where you'd planned to practice medicine, and we know that you turned down an opportunity to be rich and famous to stay here at Grady." Willetts eyed his audience. My brief trip to Hollywood was well known. "We all know that you've been working long, hard hours that must be taking their toll on your, uh, private life." He paused here to smile briefly around the table, infuriating me and bringing chuckles from everybody but Miss Ida and Beulah. Miss Ida gave Willetts a look that would freeze-dry coffee. Beulah dilated her perfect nostrils and raised her eyebrows. "All of us have the highest regard for your professional ability and we sincerely want to support the decisions you make here at Trafford, but we all feel that now is a good time to bring you a little closer to some harsh fiscal realities we're having here at the hospital."

I nodded to Willetts, determined not to lose my cool, when suddenly I felt something warm and alive crawling up the inside of my ankle, creeping up my socks and into the cuff of my trousers. Jesus! Beulah had kicked off a spiked heel pump and was doing a foot job on me in the middle of the authority board meeting.

Somebody had turned up the fan and the flypaper swirled, twisted, and snapped every third revolution of the blades.

"This hospital costs $2,000,000 a year to run. It gets $400,000 from the citizens of this county through property tax, which means it must clear about $133,333 per month on the average. Hell, Dr. Stone, we're facing a quarter million dollar shortfall this year. The county's going to advance us that amount from the money already collected for next year's budget so we can guarantee payroll, but we don't have any reserves, and they don't either. Unless we improve, something will have to be cut."

The foot in its sensual nylon skin sidled up my calf. Bound at the knee by the trouser cuff, it had pushed upward. The foot squirmed, and a toe, wiggling under the binding cloth like the probing head of a snake, tickled the inside of my knee. I nodded agreeably to Willetts. I was starting to sweat.

"We're going to need your cooperation. If we don't fix this mess, we'll have to shut the doors or the county will have to cut its health budget, and the only other choices are the ambulance service and the health department. We're all in this together, son, but you are the one calling the shots."

Beulah was lounging in her ladderback chair, her armpit hooked over the back, turned away from me at an impossible angle. She was facing Willetts, whose intermittent gaze slid to Beulah, drawn to the magnetic polarity of her cameo cleavage. Willetts was sweating too. I didn't see how a Siamese contortionist could manage what she was doing from her position, but the foot had to be Beulah's. Or Miss Ida's. Well, the foot *had* to be Beulah's.

But now it was Miss Ida's turn to speak.

"You done great things with Bill's pancreatitis, honey," she said. "We never heard of blood fat causing all his trouble. Even Carl Hogue in all those years he took care of Bill never come up with that one. I think we're obliged to give Otis more time," she told the others. The board were all in agreement about one thing: Nobody wanted to buck Miss Ida. "I can remember when Carl Hogue was a young doctor and I was a young girl. Don't many of y'all go back quite that far, but Doc Hogue probably thought of himself as a intern just like this boy does, but Doc Stone will outgrow it just like Doc Hogue did. Just let him get some more experience under his belt and we'll have a better doctor than we ever bargained for."

"He's probably got plenty of experience *under his belt*," Beulah cooed. The others, including Miss Ida, guffawed.

I squirmed in my chair, prepared to speak as the foot mercifully slithered backwards from the band of bunched trouser leg . . . only to reappear, resting now on the inside of my thigh.

"Miss Ida," I began in a voice with a noticeable bleat, caused perhaps by fluctuations in the same testosterone Shelly was worried about, "I'm an INTERNIST, not an intern. Don't you people understand that? I'm a board certified internist. The American College of Physicians has recognized my training and has declared me an ADULT MEDICINE SPECIALIST. I don't do surgery, I don't deliver babies, perform abortions, treat heartworm in dogs, see children, or do autopsies for the sheriff's department. I'll bring the best medicine I can to Trafford, but I will not exceed the limits of my expertise."

My hands were taking on a life of their own. The fingers of one hand strummed the tabletop while the other fist clenched and relaxed repeatedly as though milking an invisible cow.

"Your hospital is losing money," I continued, attempting to be assertive but betrayed by my voice, "because you don't have enough good doctors. You need at least two family physicians, a surgeon, and another internist to join me. I appreciate the sacrifices this county has made in the name of medicine, but the last thing you want to do is make a good doctor bad." My last word, altered by the removal of Beulah's foot from my thigh and its replacement on the dead center of my crotch, sounded out like the anguished call of a lamb.

"Are you aw right, doctor?" interjected a concerned Harry Defoe.

"He's losing his voice," announced Miss Ida.

"Doctor Stone's right," intoned the velvet voice of Beulah Parker, her great toe stroking, her hooded eyes sleepily amused at the degree of my involuntary response to her gentle gouging. I wished mightily for elastic trousers.

Now that Beulah faced me, Willetts stared unabashed at the tops of her breasts, mesmerized, as though he were being drawn body and soul into that formidable cleavage. Then, unbelievably, she rested a limp bejewelled wrist on Harry's shoulder, brushing his cheek with her bright fingernails as she spoke. With the other hand she tapped the table with a yellow pencil. "A physician who exceeds his comfort level isn't much of a doctor and he isn't much of a man," she said.

God, she was doing everything but calling her husband Lee Bob Parker by name. She tossed her head backwards as if to acknowledge the other members, slinging her thick black hair over her shoulder. "My father, Karl Wright, understands the predicament the hospital has gotten into. As you all know, he's done quite well managing other hospitals in the surrounding area, buying them outright and bringing them under his corporation's management. Daddy says it's just a matter of time before private corporations and the U.S. government control all the medicine in this country. Anyway, given the soft spot Daddy holds in his heart for Trafford, I believe he could be persuaded to buy the hospital, taking it off the county's hands and leaving our illustrious Dr. Stone to worry his handsome head about matters of medical concern, leaving the management of Trafford to the corporation's professionals." I remembered the *accidental* red push-pin in Wright's map and the deliberate one Beulah stuck into the lapel of my dinner jacket under the judgmental eyes of the trophy giraffe.

The details of what followed during the hospital authority meeting remain unclear. To say that sexual politics took part in what transpired would be to grossly understate, but basically I agreed to keep all the patients I could, short of compromising my ethics, which is what I was trying to do in the first place.

Without Miss Ida there I think Beulah and Willetts would have arranged a sale to Wright on the spot. They'd probably brought the papers with them. But the authority voted to pay a medical manpower search firm $25,000 to headhunt family practitioners and a surgeon. They even agreed to guarantee a half year's salary for my brother-in-law Jim Maloy, if I could get him to come to Grady. To bring in Maloy, all I had to do was convince him to sacrifice or postpone his cardiology fellowship at Emory and come to Grady as soon as he and my sister Nancy finished up their mission assignment in Guatemala. *Just put your career on hold, sports fans, and jump flat-footed into the mess I've made of my life.*

The meeting adjourned, but I remained seated a few moments. Then after the room had cleared, and I was better composed, I rushed outside to catch Beulah. I had no idea what I was going to do or say if I caught her. I burst into the bright sunlight to see her tan Mercedes roar away.

Chapter Twenty-Five

Well, did you convince Beulah Wright and the others you aren't a pedophile?" Shelly asked when I arrived home.

"What?" Guilty things start upon guilty summons. I'd still been unable to sweep away the lingering visions of Beulah. This wasn't exactly pleasant, like the way a rattlesnake you've almost stepped on keeps coming back to mind.

"A joke, Dr. Stone, a bad pun. You know, pedophile, pediatrician?"

"Oh, yes, I think I convinced them." I blinked my eyes until my mind was on Shelly. "Their problem was with *intern, internist.*"

She had grilled steak so rare and tender I imagined that mine twitched when I gigged it with my fork. To go with it, she'd prepared a squash souffle, sourdough biscuits, and Caesar salad. I enjoyed a scotch, watching the blue smoke drift from the grill and hover over Lake Loonie.

When I knew Shelly was going to be at my house, I had the satisfying sensation of coming home. She was an exciting paradox--a savvy EMT able to top the men in a men's field, yet feminine, sexy, and even domestic when the spirit moved her. I'd learned not to count on domestic.

I wondered if I'd ever be able to call Grady home, then shocked myself by realizing that I'd already begun to do just that, at least more than I'd ever thought of Washington as home. Who could be from Washington D.C. anyway? Jim Maloy, my brother-in-law, knew without a doubt where his hometown was. His diploma from Fremont's St. Joseph High School he esteemed equally with his M.D. degree from Stanford. "I'm from Fremont, Ohio," he'd say, "home of Rutherford B. Hayes. The B stands for Birchard." Then he'd plunge into a historical accounting: "In the war of 1812 young Major George Croghan with a band of 160 men repelled an invasion from a combined force of 5,000 British and Indians at Fort Stephenson on the Sandusky . . . ."

"Stop!" Nancy and I would yell in unison. "Stop with that historical bullshit!" We'd heard his monologue and other insignificant details about Fremont so many times, we could have served as tour guides if a misguided tourist ever dead-ended in Fremont. I envied Jim's easy and natural sense of who he was and where he came from. If I suddenly died of leukemia or got run over by a truck, I had no idea where my remains would be interred. Jim knew exactly where he'd be buried. Right between his father and his uncles, among three generations of Maloys, in a plot in St. Joseph's Cemetery that was already paid for. Grady, with Shelly in it, had started to give me a sense of belonging. I wondered if I should tell her.

"Why so pensive?" she asked. "Still worried about Miss Ethel's Coumadin?"

I spun her around, pulled her against me, and kissed her suddenly. She had to react quickly to avoid puncturing me with the barbecue fork.

"Whoa Doctor, let's eat supper fast. Then you can give me an anatomy lesson."

"A refresher course," I agreed.

But true to form, when I was halfway finished with my steak, the phone rang. Shelly answered it. "It's Margaret Holt for you," she said, sticking out her tongue as she handed me the receiver.

"Buster bringing in Wilkin Wright again," Margaret said.

"Send somebody to pick me up in the ambulance," I told her, hanging up. With Shelly and me both without transportation, the EMT's had to double as a taxi service. I wasn't a bit closer to being able to afford a new engine block for my Porsche. I was going to have to find another car. That's all there was to it.

"Let Flowers handle it," Shelly begged, taking my hand. "You've been out until after three a.m. for the past two nights."

"I think Flowers is strung out again," I said. "He told Margaret he had a stomach virus and was dehydrated. She has an IV going on him now in the ER annex."

"I'll clean up here and stick around," Shelly said. "Wake me up for the anatomy lesson when you get back."

Wright was comatose when I got to the ER, and Margaret was starting an IV. "Dr. Stone, we got all the stuff ready like last time."

"Wait a second with the insulin, Margaret. Something's different."

Wilkin was pale, his skin clammy. He wasn't hyperventilating and his breath didn't smell fruity from acetone. His pupils were pinpointed and he didn't budge when I raked his shinbone--perhaps a little too hard--with my reflex hammer. I caused a bruise just below his knee. I was pretty frustrated by being robbed of a rare evening with Shelly. Well, I was pissed off.

"Has anyone done a dextrose stick?" I asked Margaret.

Buster looked over at her. "I guess I forgot Wilkin's sugar always stays up. I must've brought him in five times myself with high sugar, drunk or stoned and not taking his insulin."

"Margaret, get me a D-stick stat!"

I pricked Wright's index finger with a lancet and blotted a drop of blood on a dextrose stick that gives a rough blood sugar estimate in 20 seconds. "Christ, Buster, he's a white-out. Sugar's been less than 40 for the past 20 minutes. That's why he's comatose. Margaret, give him one amp of D-50 as fast as you can push it."

I started a head and neck exam and a detailed neurologic. With alcoholic diabetics a patient can have multiple reasons for blackout, including trauma. I wanted to make sure there were no signs for increased intracranial pressure on the optic nerve. I was looking in Wilkin's left eye when he bolted upright.

"You sumbitch, get out my fuckin face!" he snarled. "I'll kill your ass!" He jumped up from the stretcher, locking my head in his right arm and smashing my jaw with his left fist. My stethoscope, caught between his biceps and my temple, pushed into my ear.

"Goddammit," I mumbled into his ribs. He hit me again, this time on top of the head.

"Buster!" cried Margaret Holt, grabbing Wilkin's hair and bending back his head.

Just as I was graying out from the strangle hold, Buster hit Wilkin like Dick Butkis flattening a quarterback. The three of us crashed through the curtain that separated Dr. Flowers from the rest of the world. We knocked him off his stretcher, and we all went down in a heap. Margaret piled on with a syringe of Valium and remarkably was able to stick it into the right combatant. Wilkin was asleep again in thirty seconds, and we were able to start crawling out of the pile-up.

Margaret still had some of Wilkin's hair she'd been holding when Buster nailed him. She wiped the remaining strands off on her apron.

Flowers was curled up like a chipmunk, shrouded in the curtain and tangled in his own IV tubes. We put him back on his stretcher and hooked him back up. "How's your virus?" I asked as Margaret re-hung the curtain over the entrance to his annex. I'd had dissected cadavers that looked better than Flowers. "Can I get you something or do you want me to call in Dr. Hooks?" He smiled weakly. I put a blanket over him and left him to his demons. The poor bastard was a bundle of bones wrapped in OR green. As soon as he leveled off, I'd talk to him about going off and drying out. Tough love.

"Thanks Buster," I croaked when we'd straightened up the ER. "You too, Margaret. I owe you both." Buster dusted off his maroon trousers.

"What the hell got into Wright, doc?" asked Buster, whose vocabulary was still growing by leaps and bounds. "He's a veritable asshole with a dysfunctional personality disorder, but I've never seen him attack a doctor before."

"Patients can act wild coming out of hypoglycemic coma after you shoot the dextrose to them," I said. "Sometimes they come up swinging. I even got punched out once by an orthopedic resident I treated when he blacked out in the Miami OR, but I've never seen anybody keep going like that for more than 20 seconds. When the sugar gets above 60, they usually settle down. I think Wilkin got high on something then forgot to eat. What we're seeing may be a combination of hypoglycemia with a drug-induced delirium." Wilkin would have to be very high on something, I thought, to be hanging around Grady after the *grinning* Hack gave him. I'd had a nightmare about Hack's hideous smile and jumped out of bed in a cold sweat. Wilkin, it turned out, hadn't come to Grady on his own volition. Buster had picked him up at Karl Wright's home, just over the county line.

I went over to the sink, spat blood, and worked my swollen jaw from side to side. I'd taken the oath of Hippocrates, but at that time I hadn't known that a dopehead son-of-a-bitch was going to rush me through a steak dinner, cheat me out of sex with a beautiful woman, try to break my jaw, and strangle me. Now I had to stay up all night saving his life. I should've let Hack scare him to death, I thought.

If I'd known then the extent of the heartbreak Wilkin Wright would cause before next spring, I sincerely think I'd have killed him myself.

I placed my hand across Buster's athletic shoulders and led him aside. Whatever malice he'd had for me when I'd first arrived in Grady seemed, since Dr. Hogue's death, to have dissipated entirely. Ironically, he'd had to play cupid to me and Shelly, shuttling us around in the ambulance or lending us his car. "Buster," I began, "You must have been a very good football player."

"I was all-state defensive tackle in high school," he said shyly. "I tried all kinds of ways to please my daddy. Football is about the only thing that worked out, the only thing I excelled in."

"He'd have been proud of you in the ER a few minutes ago. I'm more grateful than I can express through my dented trachea." I started to ask him to let Putnam pick up the emergencies in their county from now on when Wilkin Wright was concerned, but I'd wanted to clear the air about Shelly for a long time, and the moment seemed right." I acted like a carpetbagger coming to Grady and taking up with your girl," I said. "I hope there's no hard feelings."

Buster smiled, his hands shoved deep into his pockets. He shifted his weight from one long leg to the other. "Shelly's never been my girl. She's always been out of my star. All that was my daddy's doings, his progenital aspirations to make me somebody of substance."

"His what?"

"His fatherly hopes. Just like my career in neurosurgery. Hell, in twenty-eight years my only enterprise besides football's been rampant promiscuity, and that was mostly showing out for Shelly. I'm on the right track now, and I'm happy for y'all and wish you a serendipitous future together." He extended a meaty hand, warm from his pocket, which I took.

"You sure have improved your vocabulary in the last six months. Where did you find the *out of my star* stuff? *Romeo and Juliet* or Tappie Handson?"

Buster grinned. "That's not vocabulary. Mrs. Singletree made us read *Hamlet* in eighth grade English. I liked that line. Ophelia was out of Hamlet's star. Tappie may have liked it too, but everybody who ever went through the eighth grade in Grady had to memorize that line."

"Mrs. Singletree wasn't any kin to Hack, was she?"

"His own sweet mamma."

"That figures."

Our hatchet interment ceremony, as Buster would have described it, was interrupted by Rooster Bootman and two plainclothes Atlanta drug squad detectives. "Where's Dr. Frederick Flowers," they wanted to know. They cuffed him and read him his rights and waited as the IV bag dripped and collapsed, marking his final moments as a medicine man.

Chapter Twenty-Six

*B*uenos dias," I yelled through a telephone line that sounded like a culvert running under a forest fire. "Help!"

"What?"

"I need help!"

For two days, I'd been trying to put this call through to my sister Nancy and her husband in Guatemala. I knew there was no telephone at the mission hospital. American Express had to radio them to come down out of the mountains to return my call. Guatemala was Nancy's humanitarian dream, a marriage between their respective professions of social work and medicine.

Two more months of the twelve-month mission assignment remained. Then, after a short vacation, Jim was bound for a cardiology fellowship at Emory while Nancy practiced motherhood. I wasn't anxious to tell them Dr. Jeff Roberts and I had already arranged a postponement of Jim's fellowship if I could get Jim to come to Grady for another humanitarian tour.

"It's Oatsie Doats and the voice of America," I said, "reaching out from the swamps of Southwest Georgia to his little sister in the jungles of Guatemala."

"Doats! What's up? Did you knock up Shelly or did somebody die?" Nancy still sounded like she was speaking from a submarine, but I could understand her now.

"Somebody's dying, but it's just me."

"It's Otis!" I heard her tell Jim. "He says he's dying!"

I'd written them, describing in detail how my medical practice was eating me alive. They knew the fix I was in, and of course they sympathized, being two of the most important people to me in the world. "Nanny, I need you and Jim to come to Grady."

"From a jungle to a swamp?" she cried in disbelief. "I need my legs waxed and a pedicure."

"I'm serious."

She knew I was. Little sisters can read your emotional vibrations as they bounce off a satellite and run through a few thousand miles of corroded telephone cable.

"Oatsie, we *are* coming to Grady, between here and Atlanta. We'll stay with you a week or so. Atlanta can't be so very far from Grady. It's in the same state."

Atlanta's one-hundred eighty-six miles and about two-hundred years from Grady, I thought. I said: "I need you to stay twenty-four months, *Lo siento mucho*."

"I'd better put Jim on, since it's his career you want to ruin. I guess I still love you, Oatsie. Goodby."

Nancy and Jim were both impulsive. They'd become instantly enamoured the night I introduced them. Jim and I were seniors in med school at Stanford, roommates and best friends. She was starting a graduate program in social work, getting caught up in every cause and movement of the '70's from saving whales to marching with Jane Fonda at the Washington Monument. As Nanny's big brother, I'd have acidly opposed her instant liaison with anybody but Jim, but somehow it seemed natural for the two people I loved most in the world to love each other. Nancy moved in with us the next day, and she'd been with Jim ever since.

I could hear Nancy mumbling to Jim, apprising him of the situation that would force him to choose between the highly coveted cardiology fellowship with Emory's renowned Dr. Willis Hurst and bailing out a brother-in-law who'd gotten in over his head. Of course, for Jim there'd be no choice, and I knew it. He'd come to my rescue every time, disregarding personal cost and inconvenience. I felt like a double barreled asshole setting up my best friend and my sister. They both reacted to the world instinctively and were suckers for acts of love, fated for Grady as soon as I begged them for help. I *was* being selfish, but I'd never failed at anything in my life. How many times in the last weeks had I tried to bolster my deflating self-confidence by reminding myself: high school valedictorian, 3.8 in college, second in my class at Stanford, AOA honors. I wasn't about to flunk out in a small Southern hamlet, even if it meant drafting re-enforcements.

"How's it going, Numbnuts? I hear you're in a world of hurt." Jim had coined the "numbnuts" nickname one night over a jug of straw-basket Italian wine. He'd analyzed my ineptitude for situations in which the rules of competition weren't clearly spelled out. I did fine on a multiple choice exam, but when it came to winging it through unfamiliar or unprecedented situations, he surmised, I was lost and ineffectual. He blamed my "numbnuttedness" on not being from Fremont, Ohio, on not having the self-assurance of roots. Washington D.C., which wasn't even in a state, didn't count for much unless you were some kind of politician or lawyer. I knew that Maloy and Miss Ida would agreed on one thing at least. That I lacked assurance and needed a home.

"Jim, I've talked to Dr. Hurst," I began. "He says he'll hold your cardiology fellowship spot for two years if you'll come to Grady. Trafford's going to dip into the red to the tune of $300,000 this year, but they agreed to guarantee your salary. They're also paying a headhunter $25,000 to come up with two family docs and a surgeon. They're sticking their necks way out, but they're as desperate as I am."

"You've been talking to Hurst? You're connected."

"We're practically soul brothers." Jeff Roberts and cardiologist Mitchell Hoots had put in a good word for me with Hurst. I was beginning to network with Flint doctors.

"What's my cut and what are the chances you'll get some relief quicker than two years. I want to forge ahead, become a real doctor, buy a white Mercedes, join a country club, marry an R.N."

I heard Nancy hit him, *ooof*. She was large framed and athletic. Even playing, she packed a wallop.

"Your sister just busted my ass," Jim wheezed.

"You'll get thirty-five grand."

"A month?"

"No asshole, a year. And I'm afraid I've got to level with you that the chances of getting good replacements in here are slim. Grady isn't the end of the earth, but you can see it from here. You'd better count on two years."

"What about what's-his-name, uh, Flowers?"

"Dead meat. He got busted for Dilaudid, writing scripts for imaginary patients, having them filled in Atlanta. The best he can hope for is a one-year suspension, detox, and a restricted license for the future. He won't be back at Grady."

"Y'all got a Catholic church over yonder?" he asked, practicing his drawl. If I hadn't known before then they would come, I knew it now.

"St. Teresa's, a mission church that sends a priest from Flint once a month. You'll love the priest, an Irish guy from County Cork like your granddaddy. He's got an ulcer that's responding to medication. We have a nun, Sister Mary Evelyn, who visits patients at the local nursing home. I looked her up when I discovered that a Grady physician, one Lee Bob Parker, was treating her for iron deficiency anemia."

"How old is she?"

"73."

"What kind of racket are you guys up to? You should know, doctor, that post menopausal women don't have iron deficiencies."

"Well, Lee Bob's a piece of work. When I went by to see her, she couldn't say enough about how good her iron supplements were making her feel."

"Treat the symptoms and send the bill, huh?" For Maloy, doctors not totally dedicated to healing were subhuman.

"She had a malignant colon polyp that was hemorrhaging. I did a sigmoidoscopy and polypectomy." I couldn't wait to talk shop, to confer with another internist on a daily basis. "She's from Cork too," I added.

130

"From County Cork? The whole sacerdotal element up *yonder* has bad guts and hails from Cork?"

"A coincidence."

"What about the important stuff--anybody cover Notre Dame Highlights on Sunday morning?"

"There's a CBS affiliate in Tallahassee, a little fuzzy sometimes, but Lindsey Nelson's voice comes in loud and clear."

"How about bars, pubs, and other Irish dens of iniquity?"

"The county's dry. There're a couple of clubs you can brown bag your way into, and I have a friend who can flush up some pretty good stump."

"Whatever that is. See you in a couple of months. And Numbnuts . . . ."

"What?"

"Hang in there till then. And don't give Shelly the clap."

"Thanks." There was a lump in my throat, I admit it, but that night I didn't dream about the Bonsai Pipeline. I didn't dream about Hack's grin either.

Chapter Twenty-Seven

T he next day was Saturday, Miss Ethel Hargrove's 100th birthday. The picnic was on the grounds of the Tsalahatchee Baptist Church on Toa Plantation. Fortunately, the September weather was clear. A few puffy cumulus clouds with gray undersides teased the day but didn't threaten rain, which would have spelled catastrophe since there was no way the little wooden one-room church could have sheltered the multitude of Miss Ethel's family.

According to a coeval and perhaps erroneous journal entry: "The old matriarch had sired a veritable army of *chirrun*, grand-*chirrun*, and great-grand *younguns*." The difference between *chirrun* and *younguns* is not known unless verbal distinctions indicate with diluted kinship. I am beginning to understand the use of *mrs*--pronounced *mizz*--and that of *miss* applied to married women. *Ms* is not used since its pronunciation is identical to *mrs*.

Another notebook entry concerning Southern linguistic peculiarities observed:

Among Southerners, the use of the maiden prefix miss *with a married woman's first name is a designation more of respect than familiarity. It shows the world that the incidental husband has little or nothing to do with a married woman's identity. Besides the obvious subordination of employee to employer in close and long term relationships, the* miss *prefixes a married woman's Christian name when the husband is long dead, imprisoned for life, or far removed from the individual social designation of the wife. In other words, if the husband were* no count *(worthless) or if the speaker has to think twice to remember who the husband is, the* miss *will be attached to the first name. Miss Ethel's husband, for example, is long dead, but her singularity derives also from her age and monumental presence. Miss Ida is a designated* miss *by virtue of her strong individuality. Shelly would continue to be Miss Shelly even if married to me. But there are exceptions. Mrs. Singletree's status as schoolteacher would have entitled her to a titular* miss *attached to her Christian name, but she had insisted on being a* mrs, *and Mrs. Freelander, my mason's wife, will remain a* mrs *even though Thomas is destined to stay in prison until the last trumpet.*

How grand Miss Ethel was with the churchyard at her back and the brightly arrayed children, women, and men who gathered on three sides around her. How childishly proud I felt when she introduced me as her *white doctor* and announced that I had prevented her *passing*. She was seated like the Queen of Ethiopia in a wingback chair that had been placed at the edge of the little cemetery with all its plastic flowers. She had a chair brought up for me, and I sat beside her as hundreds of her progeny came to pay homage and offer presents and little tokens of love. She made me feel like a distinguished guest of honor, which was, I'd found, the hospitality rural blacks extended to displaced people. The quality that impressed me most about her clan was that the adults possessed Miss Ethel's air of quiet strength and impervious dignity--the unspoken and relentless legacy of her blood and brood. They were a people who knew who they were, whose children were clean, whose minds were educated, whose spouses were refined.

I realized that her vast family were successful because she expected them to be, and those expectations were passed on undiluted down the generations of her progeny.

"You want to say something, Big Mamma?" inquired one of her grandsons, a Bibb County judge who acted as M.C.

"You know I does," she said. "A woman don't live a hundred years without having something to say." She stood up, supporting herself with her walker, refusing my help and her grandson's.

"I look around here and I see my family I'm proud of," she began, nodding a head orbed by thin fleece. "My peoples has been down a long dirt road, and we ain't to the hardtop yet. I don't recollect all your names, but I knows your blood, and I can tell you this: Be strict with your children and love them because they my children too. Be patient with them because you live long enough, you'll see patience and love's the same thing. Help them fine out who they *are* and they'll learn for themselves what they want to be." She gripped the sides of her walker like a lectern and smiled. "Don't you never, never let them think you don't expect the best from them, and that's ever bit of all I has to say."

One other white man besides me had come by to pay his respects. Robert McCormick Jones, owner of the land Miss Ethel's family had occupied since before the Civil War--the land that had been owned by Wrights during slavery, when Karl Wright's forbears had owned Miss Ethel's grandparents. Mr. Mack, I discovered, hadn't displaced a single family since his acquisition of Toa, and he'd allowed former tenants displaced by his predecessors to return to the land of their ancestry. For Miss Ethel's birthday he'd personally delivered one hundred chickens fried in the kitchen of his mansion at Toa. He'd left before I had a chance to meet the eccentric philanthropist and soft drink magnate whose theme was preservation, who seemed to share the Southerners' common distrust for the implicit virtue of change.

Chapter Twenty-Eight

The eight weeks between my call to Jim and Nancy and their arrival were the most stressful I'd ever experienced. Shelly had moved in, more a supportive gesture than romantic since I was more often than not too tired to argue about what our lives had become, much less make love. I found myself tiptoeing shoeless into the old farmhouse late at night, dreading that creaking board in the floor that would wake her to love or argument, neither of which I had the energy to engage.

If I'd had the leisure to do it, I could have measured the degradation of my love life by the parade of uneaten meals Shelly prepared and left for me. The first dishes that spoiled while waiting for me to get home at reasonable hours were elaborately prepared and wholesome. They were special meals, sprinkled with paprika and trimmed with parsley--souffles, quiches, and wonderful wild game dishes with sauces of sherry or tarragon. They were the specialties of Southern cuisine which Shelly, of course, knew how to cook well although she ate animal flesh sparingly.

Gourmet cuisine regressed into simpler dishes that would keep--soups, casseroles, stews, gumbos--healthful mixtures that could be reheated or even carried in a thermos to the office or hospital. The next food I found when I dragged in after midnight had atrophied into sustenance that was neither particularly nutritious nor appetizing. This was the Italian period, when I'd find a mound of cold spaghetti, a lump of leftover lasagna, or a wedge of rubbery pizza. During the Italian period I'd drag in during the predawn hours with a billy goat's worth of B.O. under each arm. I'd be too exhausted to shower and too malodorous to pollute the prenuptial bed. I'd drop dead on the couch and try to snatch two or three hours sleep before time to get up, rinse off, and rush back to the relentless battle against the diseases and catastrophes of the poor.

The poor didn't often pay in barter as they had in the days of Carl Hogue's youth, but they paid slowly and often brought fruit, produce, and poultry for good will or accrued interest on payments long in arrears. Two notable exceptions to the prohibition against barter were Syndrome, the sow that wound up incarcerated with Hack's daddy in the electrified junkyard, and a fighting game cock, Napalm, which was reputed to be worth $500 to everybody but me.

The chicken, bright as a blacksmith's hearth, was also adopted by Hack and Melvin Dryden, who strengthened the cock's wings by throwing it repeatedly against a barn. They developed its legs by holding it in a squat and running it back and forth along a plank. Soon they alchemically transmuted the rooster into a rebuilt transmission for a serviceable Ford Falcon, since Melvin had finally pronounced my red Porsche beyond repair. Hack warned that if Shelly found out that the Falcon was vaguely connected to cockfighting, she wouldn't set her *cloven* ass on the upholstery.

Luckily, since I didn't have time to eat the food my patients brought me, I was able to work out a system of credits and exchange with the grocer, Glen Aborotie, who let me "*swap out*" some of the produce for cash or credit in his store. I had more money than I could spend because I didn't have time to spend money.

Looking back with 20/20 hindsight, I can see that dark and hectic period with clarity and perspective. These were the weeks that encompassed the hopeless lingering on of the hospital and the clinic, my marrow-deep exhaustion and self doubt, my leeched and eroded love affair with Shelly. I was pushing myself beyond my ability to succeed. If I hadn't enjoyed the hope of reinforcement from the Maloys, I'd have spontaneously combusted and burned entirely out. Of course, my assurance that help would come may have prevented me from setting a more reasonable pace. "When there's dead fish on your trotline and you run over your dog," Hack told me, "it means you ain't in the groove." I didn't know what he meant at the time, but later I did. My tragic flaw of ignoring my instincts, again, was at the root of my ineptitude as a physician and lover. I was not practicing what Dr. James Maloy would later jokingly term the *art of Zen and community medicine.*

A grim point in fact was the case of George Washington Hawkins, a tall eighty-three-year-old black man whose sinewy frame had been sculpted by a life of hard physical labor divided between dirt farming and pulpwood operations. I first attended him when he amputated a finger with a chain saw. He came into the clinic, the stump of his index finger wrapped in a turpentine poultice. There was little I could do except block a digital nerve to relieve the pain and treat him for infection, but Mr. Hawkins was grateful to the extent of sending me a multitude of patients from his considerable progeny. Under my care, however, George died of a subdural hematoma--a blood clot in the brain.

Chapter Twenty-Nine

When I saw the Maloys disembark the airplane, I was happy beyond my ability to express it. The runway wind blew Nancy's Guatemalan dress against her strong legs and lashed her hair as she walked confident and tall toward the terminal. Jim followed with his self-assured smile. "Here they come!" I told Hack, expecting him to pick them out from all others.

"I reckon they are," laughed Hack. "Everybody's off the plane but the pilot and the stews. But I know which two belong to you. They ain't but two Yankees the right age to be the Maloys." He pointed them out correctly, and I wasn't surprised. They were strong and tan with eyes that sparkled with health and enthusiasm. There wasn't anything I couldn't accomplish with those two here. "Nanny! Jimbo!" I called, waving.

"Oatsie!" Nancy ran, hugging me, nearly knocking me down. "This must be Hack," she said, kissing his cheek. Then Maloy was there, shaking Hack's hand, slapping him on the shoulder, giving me a bear hug.

"You're a *physical* bastard," I smiled.

"Hello Numbnuts," said Maloy.

We loaded the Maloys' earthly possessions into the bed of Hack's pickup and squeezed into the cab. Nancy and Jim were ravenous for Chinese, having been denied it for two years at the mission. Hack insisted on buying. "Just put enough of whatever you're cooking in some cartons," he told the waitress, "enough for about ten of us. Melvin's got Daddy," he explained, "and we can run some by to Shelly and Buster." Hack was always thoughtful of Shelly. Then he told the diminutive Oriental proprietor he wanted extra orders of grits and kimchi.

"No hobba grits," the woman said. "This Chinee place."

"Come on, Hack," I said. "Leave the Chinese lady alone. Let's go get a bottle of Irish whiskey to celebrate the arrival of these illustrious Micks."

"Hell, she ain't Chinese," Hack said. "She's Korean or I'm a A-rab. What you think a Chinese gal's doing with kimchi? But I *heard* that about the whiskey."

The girl came back with another carton, grinning wide enough, as they say in the vernacular, to cut the top of her head off.

"*Ko-map-sum-nee-dah,*" Hack told the girl.

"*Chum-an-nay-o,*" she answered, bright-eyed and grinning up at Hack, who seemed nearly twice her height.

"Where'd you learn how to speak Korean?" I asked. "I didn't know you'd ever been out of Georgia."

"Uncle Sam sent me over yonder on a military fellowship."

"You didn't write me that your friend Hackamore was a world traveler,"

Nancy said.

"I didn't know it myself," I told her.

"Let's get over to that liquor store," Hack said.

Whatever we had in the bags and cartons filled the cab of the pickup with mouth-watering aroma, and we ate the egg rolls on the way to the liquor store. "Get some wine and beer," said Nancy. "I don't know if we should drink the water down South."

"I wouldn't," Hack grinned.

"He doesn't," I confirmed.

We went to Lake Loonie where we ate and drank merrily, telling old stories, recalling childhood and med school memories. Solving world problems, saving Grady and Guatemala. I felt as though a high pressure area had just blown in from the west and cleared a cloudy and oppressive horizon of my future. There was nothing I couldn't do. I was rescued, imbued with new life. Like a spring snake that's just crawled out of his old skin.

Then Shelly called and the curtain fell.

"We just brought George Hawkins in," she said, "D.O.A."

Mrs. Hawkins had brought George in just before Hack and I went to the airport. Hawkins complained of a headache, the *wust* one he'd ever had, said Mrs. Hawkins. The patient answered *Yessuh* to every question I asked him. I made a quick examination of his scalp and made sure he could flex and extend his neck. I had him walk on his toes and checked his balance. "Lordy, Lordy, Lordy," he said suddenly. "Lordy, Lordy, Lordy, Lordy." Finding no obvious cause for his pain, I gave Mrs. Hawkins a head trauma sheet and told her to call me if any of the categorized symptoms developed. In my hurry to dismiss them and rush to the airport to pick up the Maloys, I overlooked the clue that could have saved the old man's life. What I should have paid strict attention to were his *tachylordias*, a diagnostic sign unique to the deep South.

Hawkins was, except for Dr. Hogue (who refused to follow orders) my first patient to expire, and I felt responsible. My ignorant adherence to the rules killed him. I'd treated the patient like a multiple choice quiz, and he failed to comply, dying.

Chapter Thirty

The music, surpassing all other gospel singing I'd ever heard, was passionate, loud, and strangely beautiful, in profound contradiction to the ecclesiastical music of my Catholic childhood. I could actually feel the tingling vibration of the pews against my buttocks and the backs of my thighs. The stained windows rattled. "We're gone cross that river Jordan," we sang. "We be there together on the other side." The collective body of the choir swayed as powerful song and joyful noises reverberated through the air and stirred it to heavy palpability--air that couldn't be breathed into the lungs without infecting them with song. It wasn't music that began in voices and fell on ears. It was a tremulous, spiritual anthem that flowed through us--mad, wonderful music that amalgamated the singers into a fluid, tingling oneness of spirit. I was reminded of the vibrant heat I felt when I touched the snake-eye disk in Hack's study. I was possessed briefly by powerful metaphysical sensations that made my whiteness, my education, my gender, my national origin absolutely irrelevant. I was moved, stunned, and very nearly frightened.

After the music, I settled down some, holding back as the congregation participated in the eulogy, hearing the amens, the hallelujahs, the short testimonials, the final words from friends and neighbors and finally from George's pastor, who spoke with the dramatic, ministerial rhetoric I'd noticed typical of blacks--preachers, lawyers, funeral directors, politicians--when speaking to audiences.

There were many flowers, each arrangement held up individually by Stokes, the funeral director himself, who wore a tuxedo with tails. He announced the contributors to an audience, who hummed and sighed in appreciation.

"Doctor Otis Stone and his associates at Grady Medical Health Care Clinic," Stokes said, panning my wreath before the congregation. My name sounded as foreign to me as Arabic.

Hack and I had been the only whites in the little wooden country church. The pine floors creaked as we were ushered to our position of honor near the open coffin. I felt that I'd been placed in plain view of the corpse so that I might consider my sin and shoulder the ponderous burden of my contrition. I wouldn't have been much surprised if George Hawkins had sat up in his silk-lined coffin and pointed the amputated stump of his index finger at me proclaiming my guilt.

I was astonished by the open emotion of the congregation--the wailing and moaning, the screams of family, the grief responses--and they made me feel indeed like a visitor in a strange land. I was alarmed when Mrs. Hawkins stood up, raising her arms into the air. "O George!" she cried. "Why you leave me here alone? You know I cain make it on this here Earth by myself!" She shook with sobbing.

Two women, dressed in starched white nursing uniforms and capes, rushed to her side, embracing her, petting, and whispering.

"Oh, let me go on with him!" Mrs. Hawkins cried. "Let me PASS!" Others cried out. A few swooned and were attended to in turn. Some fell to their knees on the floor, where they sobbed and raved. I could feel myself being moved. My eyesight blurred, and I found a lump in my throat.

"Is this the way it's usually done?" I asked Hack out of the side of my mouth. "I've got to get out of here."

His head was down and his lips were moving, as in silent prayer. He'd read the bulletins and tithe envelopes and was working on the hymnal. He looked up. "No you ain't," he hissed, marking his place with a thick finger. "You got to stay right where you're at."

"The nurses?" I whispered. "Are the nurses always there?" For some reason the presence of nurses made me feel doubly damned. As though my blunder had carried over to jeopardize the survivors.

"Always," Hack's rasped.

"R.N.'s?"

"Course not. This look like a hospital to you?"

At the end of the service, the congregation passed in single file past the coffin, some speaking to George, some touching his coffin. "I'm sorry," I told him as I passed by.

"Whew! That wrung me out," I said when we were back at Hack's truck.

"It's supposed to," Hack said. "Black funerals pull it out of you. White funerals ain't nothing beside a black funeralizing. You want to go to Crown Hill and see old George go in the ground?"

"No, I think I've had enough. I almost broke down in there. I guess it's because I still feel responsible. . . .I killed him," I said. I'd already told the Maloys and Shelly about my screw-up, but something--culpability, I guess--made me need to confess to a layman.

"Naw. You go to a black funeral, you feel like that. You get the notion that we're all in this thing together."

"What thing?"

"The trip from down here to over yonder. When somebody gets funeralized proper, you feel the vacuum sucking when you turn him a-loose."

"No man's an island?"

"There you go."

I became emotional because I felt guilty, although Hack wasn't willing to buy that *load of horseshit*. "You feel guilty? That some Catholic hoodoo or what? I thought Jews was the ones big on guilt." He waited until most of the people had dispersed or joined the procession before he cranked the truck, which gasped, rumbled, and emitted white flatulence. I watched the smoke drift into the old tombstones and markers, many of them made of Savannah brick. Slaves were often buried under Savannah brick. The little graveyard beside the church was full, bulging at the seams. George Hawkins would be buried in a new cemetery, nine miles away.

"No. It doesn't have anything to do with religion. I ignored pertinent information in establishing probabilities around Hawkins' differential diagnosis."

"You what? I hope you don't talk like that on top of Shelly."

I'd been excited about meeting Jim and Nancy at the airport and I'd ignored my gut feeling to hospitalize Hawkins. My training had taught me to ignore gut feelings, to be objective, and that's what I'd done, causing Hawkin's death.

Hack pulled out on the highway, going the opposite direction of the slow procession. "Differential Diagnosis!" he grinned, shifting into second as the old truck backfired and complained.

"Think about a murder investigation," I explained. "Rooster Bootman would establish a list of suspects."

"Yeah, Rooster would get to the scene of the crime, kicking ass and taking names."

Through a rusted out spot in the floorboard I could see the highway whizzing beneath us. "Well, a good internist integrates clues from the medical history, physical exam, and lab work to establish probable causes for a given ailment. Then he comes up with a list of suspects, his differential diagnosis. If one of the suspects poses an immediate threat, he arrests the illness by hospitalizing the patient."

Hack was delighted by what he called my utopian view of science with its endless metaphoric applications. To my cosmography he added a metaphor of his own: "A happy hog walks nut-deep in pigshit." Although I wasn't 100% sure what he meant, I gathered he didn't have much faith in the infallibility of a differential diagnosis.

I'd done a technically flawless neurological exam on Hawkins. There was no blood behind his eardrums, indicating major trauma. I examined his fundi with the ophthalmoscope, the lighted instrument that allows us to see the optic nerve, which is actually a little part of the brain tissue. A bulge indicates pressure on the brain. I listened to the neck vessels for bruits--noises that indicate a blood vessel is blocked--and I examined the neck to make sure it was not stiff or inflexible from meningitis or a broken bone. I related the procedure to Hack.

". . . and the patient dropped dead, so you're just sad," he said. "I love it when you talk doctor, but you *ain't* guilty. The autopsy said George died of a blood clot in his noodle. Your only clue was a headache. Hell, I got a headache right now. He could've been out the night before drinking bad stump."

"No, the *lordies*, the *tachylordias*, should have alerted me that the clot was ripping up his brain while I examined him."

"*Tachylordia* don't sound like something you learned in med school. It ain't nowhere near as classy as *differential diagnosis.*

Hogue, Holt, Shelly, and the other EMT's had coined a frivolous term for a serious symptom. *Tachylordias* worked like a Buddhist chant, a mantra, putting religious patients in touch with their pain and their maker. If the patient whispers "lordy" fewer than, say, ten times a minute, the pain's not severe, indicating perhaps the flu or a urinary tract infection, for example. Shelly calls this *bradylordia*, but Hawkins had *tachylordias* twice in my office, a rapid repetition of *lordy* as he clutched his head between his palms. The key to this case was that I ignored the new onset of severe headache, which called for a differential diagnosis of: *new onset "worst headache of life."* The differential suspects then would be: ruptured intracranial aneurysm, subdural hematoma, meningitis, and a few minor pathologies, but the first three can kill.

I should have hospitalized George instead of sending him home with a head sheet nobody in the family could read. Hawkins had begun vomiting when he got home. He became lethargic and his left pupil dilated. His eighty-year-old wife could have followed his neurologic progression. If she'd been able to read, she could have seen that his prognosis indicated imminent coma and death. Even after missing my chance to hospitalize George, I'd presumed Mrs. Hawkins could read a head sheet. That was sheer stupidity, I now realized.

"What *is* a head sheet?" Hack, possibly the best-read resident of Grady County, asked.

The October landscape crawled by--the farmland's tawny stubble, the flamboyant reds and yellows of the hedgerows and canebrakes and woods. The road skirted the east edge of the Swamp of Toa, and I noticed the cypress of creek banks and bottoms were fringed with gold. Nearly every truck I'd see from now until January would have a deer rifle or shotgun in the rear window rack--a sight which would cause Shelly in passing to hiss, sputter, and curse.

"What are the odds in this county of an eighty-year-old rural black woman being able to read a head sheet?" I asked Hack.

"Not good," he admitted. "She'd of been born around the turn of the century. There wasn't a lot of educational opportunity around here for country folks during the first decade of the 1900's, especially if you happened to be black. But don't fret. The Hawkins family ain't the type to sue for malpractice."

"That's not the point. My records reflect impeccable work. No lawyer, not even Delmore Abalone, would touch this case." Abalone was an Atlanta attorney who specialized in improbable malpractice suits. I'd get a ten on technical merit.

I flunked out--not in science, but in art. "Shelly keeps saying I practice medicine like an academic competition where the AOA pin goes to the quiz show champ. She says I'll make a doctor when I jump off the ivory tower of my med school professors and land on my 'cleft ass' upon the red clay of Grady County, Georgia, U.S.A. She says I'll be a community's doctor when I'm a part of a community, not an academic appendage."

"Maybe Shelly's too hard on you," Hack said. "Maybe you're being too hard on yourself. You live, you learn. Everybody's dying. The last census showed more dead folks than live ones already, and the dead ones keep on piling up. You liable to outlive a lot of patients. If you drag ass feeling guilty every time somebody dies, you ain't gone be worth steer shit in a cattle drive. Shelly's a right smart girl. You stay with her. You'll be aw right."

It amused me that Hack never missed an opportunity to defend Shelly. Although she had mellowed some in her animosity, she was never far away from verbally blistering his ass. Hack was old enough to be her father, but she treated him with a contemptuous familiarity which polite Southerners usually reserve for contemporaries. She must have rebelliously opposed her parents in her girlhood infatuation for Hack. When they died, she came to hate him in their honor. The truck rattled into the parking lot of the clinic. Mr. Freelander, on one knee beside his grandson, smiled and waved.

"She's right, Doc," Hack said. "A man ain't whole till he's part of something bigger than his Oldsmobile. Forget the research center and the white rats. Stay right here in Grady, where you can practice real medicine on *real* folks. Poor folks hurt just as bad as rich ones do."

———————

I learned another important lesson that October from one Virginia Pitman, a seventy-eight-year-old widow of a veteran killed in the first assault of Okinawa. Miss Virginia taught me that high spirits, pride, and impeccable appearance do not necessarily evidence economic solvency. Miss Virginia's Southern cooking and 320 cholesterol occluded 90% of her left main coronary artery. When Inderal caused depression, I switched her to a new beta-blocker Tenormin, which was reported to cause less depression. I didn't realize that this drug cost $78-a-month and that she would make the near-fatal choice of not filling the prescription. She had full Medicare, an Army widow's pension, and a Social Security check of $386 a month, but she had children and grandchildren she didn't want to depend on or neglect. She bore the secret of her financial destitution as faithfully as she remained true to the memory of her dead husband. I ended up having to send her to Putnam's Jeff Roberts with a whopping anterior infarct. After I got her shipped, I found a three-month supply of Tenormin samples left by the drug rep.

From then on I became known among drug companies as a con man of expensive medication samples. Since Miss Virginia I made a point to know what the drugs I prescribed cost and whether that expense was going to prevent my patient's taking the prescribed amount.

Chapter Thirty-One

I knew Dr. Paul Dudley, District Health Director of Southwest Georgia, was an aficionado scattergun marksman, so I asked him to invite me to the Tailfeathers Skeet and Trap Club one October Sunday. I wanted to pick his brain for suggestions on how to get Federal funding for Grady as an underserved area. I wanted Maloy there, and Hack said we'd go in his truck since the Falcon was predictably at Melvin's having the carburetor overhauled. We'd planned on going to Tailfeathers after a picnic lunch in my backyard on Loonie Lake.

But it was one of those beautiful fall days when you are immortal and the sky is bright and blue as fine porcelain. Mary Lou Jackson, one of the new teachers Hack "cut from the herd," fried the chicken, the most delicious any of us had ever eaten. To go with the potato salad, deviled eggs, and garlic bread, Shelly made a blueberry cheesecake with fresh berries, and Nancy fixed a banana cake, heavy and moist, like the ones she and I remembered from our childhood in Washington. Hack brought a pint jar of mayhaw jelly. Mayhaws, he said, grew on thorny trees in the Swamp of Toa. "You've heard of Hawthornes, as in Nathaniel," Nancy said.

"I get it," said Mary Lou. We'd all liked Mary Lou immediately. When she and Hack arrived in his pickup and he'd helped her out, she looked so small we thought he'd brought a child. She had a tight, serious face and a scratchy voice. When introduced, she half-squatted in a sort of curtsy, "Pleased to make y'all's acquaintance, I'm sure," she said. She was adorable--petite, acrobatic, and childishly proportioned, except for her breasts. Like Shelly, she'd been a cheerleader in college.

Maloy raved about her fried chicken until Mary Lou satisfied him by explaining the difference in the chickens her grandmother raised and the ones wrapped in supermarket cellophane. "These chickens was yard chickens," she said, "free to scratch and roam. They picked out what they ate their ownselves and roosted in trees." Supermarket poultry, she informed us, was raised in cages and fed food pellets and chemicals. "City chickens' feet never touch the ground."

"That's been your problem, Stone," Shelly said. "Your feet never touch the ground."

"You know, you're *right*!" squealed Nancy. That's *true*! Otis has never been what you could call down-to-earth."

Hack guffawed, spilling beer in his lap, and Maloy laughed in his rich Irish way, flipping a spoonful of potato salad across the blanket, spattering my shirt.

"Food fight! Food fight!" Nancy laughed. "Otis, remember the nuns when we were kids?" We both held out our palms and winced, recollecting the punishment the nuns inflicted with rulers one day in the lunchroom of the Catholic school.

144

I had flipped an English pea at Nancy with my thumb and index finger when the good sisters' backs were turned. Nancy retaliated by slinging a forkful of tapioca pudding, some of which spattered the back of Sister Lucy's habit.

"I might have become a brain surgeon had it not been for that day when Sister Lucy transformed these prodigious hands into paws," I said dramatically.

"No food fights with these vittles," said Maloy, who lay supine, his fingers laced across his temporarily protuberant belly.

There's nothing to give a man a sense of comfort and well-being like a belly full of beer, saturated fats, and cholesterol. Our caloric intake had been astronomical, but nothing, we rationalized, could be bad for you that tasted so good.

"I've done told you," snapped Mary Lou, "there wasn't nothing added to that food."

"What do you teach, Mary Lou?" I asked her.

"English, geography, and civics."

I guess because of our mutual contentment, our sense of well being, and togetherness, when time came to go to the skeet club, the women decided they would go with us, which meant taking the ambulance instead of Hack's truck. Given Shelly's dislike of firearms *and* Hack, she surprised me by going. "How long do you have to parboil skeets," she joked, "to make them tender?" She was making a heroic effort to be civil to Hack too, as though with Mary Lou present, she was willing to release her animosity and give over to another woman the responsibility to reform Hack and put him in his place.

Hack, Mary Lou, and Maloy climbed into the back. Shelly, Nancy, and I rode in the cab. We knew if Shelly got a call, some of us would be stranded, but we reasoned that I could ride to the emergency and the others could hitch a ride to Hack's truck.

"I never been in an ambulance but once," said Mary Lou, "and that was when Bigdaddy got kicked by a cow. I had to ride in with him to make sure he didn't jump out. Bigdaddy never liked cars, much less one with a bed in the back and the kind that carries your coffin."

We arrived at Tailfeathers, hearing the muffled pops of shotguns as shooters fired at round ceramic targets that sailed through the air, breaking, transforming to black dust, or landing unscathed. Hack yelled through the crawl space to the cab for Shelly to sound the siren, but she wouldn't. Still, when we pulled up to the lodge, the ambulance caused plenty of commotion. Shooters, bunched up at the stations of all three ranges, stopped firing and glanced around apprehensively to see who had fallen out or dropped dead.

Shelly and I were used to such responses. Our arrival in the ambulance to any populated area brought bystanders a reminder that disaster is a constant in the human condition, just as the arrival of a hearse serves its spectators as a harbinger of mortality. Maloy and I had noticed, incidentally, at big city cocktail parties that stylish ladies discovering themselves in the presence of a physician unconsciously placed the palm of an elegant hand over a breast they feared might host a tumor. In Grady, where people were inclined to withhold "personal" information, reading body language became essential.

Even before I spotted Dr. Paul Dudley, I saw Dr. Country Trulane, impeccably dressed in a fawn cashmere sweater over a two-hundred dollar shooting jacket with leather patches on shoulders and sleeves. A paisley scarf was tied around his neck, and an expensive Purdey over-and-under shotgun was broken over the crotch of his elbow. He, like most of the other participants, wore amber shooting glasses and earplugs.

In contrast to the others, our group was conspicuously hodgepodge, the only gun among us being Hack's disreputable .12 gauge pump--rust-spattered and silvered--the blueing worn almost entirely from its long barrel.

Dr. Paul Dudley stepped over from a huddle of shooters, smiling amiably, shaking hands with Maloy, bowing his head to the ladies. Mary Lou half squatted in curtsey.

"I've reserved us the far range in case you want to get acquainted with the sport or in case the ladies care to shoot," Dudley said. "There's a group on the trap range who'd be honored if Hack would join them in some trapshooting. They'll shoot stickbirds later in the afternoon." Stickbirds, I'd learned, was a contest made more competitive by handthrowing the ceramic saucer-shaped targets. The contestants' skill in slinging the targets from the long-handled catapult provided greater speed and variation than did the trap and skeet throwing machines.

Hack grinned, "You got a twenty, Doc?"

"Of course not."

Maloy plundered his wallet and handed Hack a twenty-dollar bill.

"Excuse me, then," Hack said wandering off.

"I can't believe you gave him twenty dollars to throw away gambling," I told Maloy.

"Hack's not gambling," Dudley smiled. "Those other gentlemen are." Then I remembered some community outrage when Hack was accused of betting school funds at a stickbird match. He answered school board officials that betting on himself at a stickbird match was more like investing school money in a high interest blue chip stock. There had always been considerably more money in the kitty after his investments of school money than before, but if anybody didn't like the way he was operating Grady Junior High, they could step up right now and take over as principal. When nobody did, he softened, promising those present that he wouldn't wager school monies on dog or chicken fights, cards or craps, or any endeavors where there was an element of chance. He also promised he wouldn't even shoot stickbirds if he ever got too drunk to hit the ground with his hat. And he would not shoot live pigeons at all, except in the direst fiscal emergency, out of respect for the county's more sensitive citizenry.

Dudley led us to a semicircle of concrete bases with a low rectangular "house" on one end and a taller one on the other, which were called the low and high houses respectively. Shooters, changing positions from one base to the next, called for targets to be thrown from each house. Skeet differed from trap in that trap shooters stood behind a bunker from which the clay targets were thrown.

Dudley released clay pigeons from the houses by pushing buttons on an apparatus that looked like a remote control TV channel changer on a long electrical cord. A metal arm slung the ceramic disc--*ther-whacka-wack*--from the high house window. It sailed quickly, hovered, then dropped, breaking as it dropped to the ground some fifty yards out.

"We'll shoot the highhouse bird from the number seven station," Dudley said, "until you get the feel of the gun. Then we'll shoot the lowhouse bird. Later, if you feel like it, we'll shoot a round." Paul Dudley was a lean, grandfatherly man in his sixties, with aviator glasses and thin gray hair combed back. An epidemiologist in khaki trousers and tweed coat, Dudley was public health director of the fourteen-county district that encompassed southwest Georgia.

He helped us choose shotguns from a gun rack, fitting us by placing the stock in the crotch of our elbows and having us reach the trigger with our index fingers. After he'd found a fit for everybody but Mary Lou, he identified our dominate eye by having us look through a circle made at arm's length by touching index fingers to thumbs. Our dominate eye was the one that lined up a distant object in the circle from the same angle as the object lined up with both eyes open. This was to know whether we should shoot right handed or left.

He left us practicing, pointing empty guns at an empty sky, while he walked across the range for a conference with Harry Defoe, whom I'd met on the hospital authority. Harry had sawed off the stock of a .28 gauge doublebarrel for his son's ninth birthday. He kept the gun behind the seat of his pickup for snakes or in the unlikely event that he'd find an enthusiastic child with an overindulgent parent who'd buy it. When Harry discovered that Mary Lou needed a smaller gun, his eyes brightened. He hurried over with the .28 gauge and a half dozen boxes of shells.

We beginners stayed on the seventh station, situated immediately in front of the low house, so that targets thrown from the high house sailed toward us. Low house birds flew almost directly away. Dudley told us the seventh station was considered the best to learn on. "It's not necessary to lead targets flying straight toward a shooter or straight away," he explained. Leading meant shooting in front of a target to compensate for its speed.

I shot first at a highhouse target, the target sailing unscathed over my head as the 12 gauge over-and-under jarred my shoulder and rattled my molar fillings. "Hold the butt snug against your shoulder," Dudly advised. "The gun will kick you if you don't." Shelly hit her "bird" on her second try, and Maloy dusted his first target and continued to shoot with the effortless grace he had for everything he tried. Nancy shot only slightly better than I did, hitting about one out of five of the targets.

But it was Mary Lou who surprised us by shooting nearly as well as Maloy and taking to skeet shooting with a passion. "Sling me another one of them suckers, Paul Dudley," she sang out in her scratchy voice. "I'm hot as a two-dollar pistol!"

"Shall I serve you up a double, Miss Mary Lou?" said Dr. Dudley after a quarter hour of instruction, visibly pleased that we were having fun.

"Send 'em on out yonder," squealed Mary Lou, and he pressed the doubles button. Targets sailed from both houses. "Yahoo!" she cried, powdering one bird and chipping the other. "This is more fun than breaking dishes!"

As the others enjoyed themselves, I pulled Dr. Dudley aside and picked his mind for insights into the catastrophic state of affairs I was experiencing while trying to practice medicine in Grady. I told him about the hospital, the impossible numbers of patients who showed up for treatment--so many that Maloy and I found ourselves treating acute illnesses rather than practicing good comprehensive medicine that emphasized prevention.

Dr. Dudley listened patiently to me as he watched the shooters, releasing their targets with the remote control. "Start with a needs assessment," he said. "I'll help you with it. Find out who your patients are and what kinds of health problems they have. Then you can establish a working relationship with your county health department to refer some of your problems to them, reducing your work load."

Maloy sensed Dudley and I were talking shop. He unloaded his gun, leaned it into the gun rack, and joined us. Before long Nancy wandered over. Her ears perked up at the first mention of public health, and she stayed. Shelly, the first to lose interest in skeet shooting, had wandered up to the clubhouse. Mary Lou alone was left at the shooter's station, "Pull me one, Dr. Paul! Send that sucker into the *air*!"

Dudley launched a high house target, which Mary Lou cleanly missed. He handed me the remote control and walked over to instruct his prize pupil. "You're lifting your head," I heard him tell her. "You have to keep your cheek on the stock so your gun shoots where you're looking. Start with your gun pointed just about there." He wrapped his arms around her, helping her point the shotgun. "Then you've got to catch up to the bird and swing through." Mary Lou shifted her feet excitedly. "Pull!" said Paul Dudley. I pressed the button, and Mary Lou blasted the target. "That's just it, young lady," Paul said, patting Mary Lou's back. "That's just about perfect."

Paul Dudley left Mary Lou to return to his health care tutorial. "You use the health department for preventative care, reducing your daily work load so you and Dr. Maloy can concentrate on acute and chronic disease management."

"Divide and conquer?" asked Maloy, who'd placed both hands in his hip pockets and was leaning toward Dudley.

Dudley nodded. "There wasn't a finer physician in the state," he continued, "than Carl Hogue. He could do anything. But he tried to do *everything*, and he turned no one away who needed his help. He died broke and exhausted. There was an array of programs that could have helped him, but he was just like a lot of doctors in this country. He was fighting a lonely war when he should have been recruiting allies."

The Maloys were taking in every word, *pointing* Dudley, as Hack would say, like a couple of liverspot bird dogs. I was interested too. I was inexperienced, but I knew enough to realize that we were already in over our heads, that we couldn't provide quality health care to the overwhelming numbers who needed our help. If Dudley couldn't help us, at least he could sympathize. If he had a straw, I was willing to grasp it.

Soon we were seated around a sturdy picnic table used during tournaments for score keeping and supporting trophies and ammunition. Shelly had rejoined us. "When you're up to your ass in alligators," she said, "it's hard to remember you're in there to drain the swamp."

"Very well put, young lady. Almost no country physicians pool their resources effectively with public health services. They act separately, overlapping in some areas, mutually excluding others."

"Why's that?" asked Shelly.

"Yeah, why?" said Nancy.

"One thing," smiled Paul Dudley, "interaction with public health care smacks of socialized medicine, the 'S' word every American physician only whispers under cover of darkness. But a better reason, perhaps, is that cooperating with public health service means having to take a larger number of indigent patients, and that's murder on private practice. Most doctors accept charity cases, but it's their paying patients who keep their practice solvent and offset the indigent patients. The insured patients and the ones with money have to make up for the elderly and the poor."

"Charity don't pay malpractice insurance," said Jim Maloy, practicing his

Southern accent.

"Of course, you gentlemen don't have to worry about the balancing ratio of paying to indigent patients. Correct me if I'm wrong," smiled the public health director, "but I'd venture to guess that practically *all* of your patients already *are* charity. The patients in your service area who can afford to pay will commute twenty-five miles to Flint, where they don't have to wait in line alongside the untouchables. I hate to be a prophet of doom, but there's no way you're going to be able to keep doing what you're doing and keep your doors open for long. In an economic sense, you young fellows have, as the saying goes, shot craps in New Orleans."

"How'd he know?" Maloy asked me.

"I know your area, and I know you're not turning anybody away," Dudley continued. "Your service area is a textbook example of rural poverty in the South. The people you treat don't have the money to pay for your services, and many of them don't qualify for Medicare or Medicaid. Listen, 40% fall below the poverty level; half your people over 25 haven't graduated from high school; there's a 30% illiteracy rate. This state has the highest infant mortality rate in the nation, and Grady County has the highest infant mortality in the state. *And* not surprisingly, the highest teen pregnancy rate. Jesus! Otis, for every 1000 girls who go through their teens in Grady County, 450 produce babies. Last year 10 babies were born to children from 10-14 years old."

"Babies having babies," said Shelly. "You're a long way from doing boob jobs for starlets at two grand a whack."

"You've got a lot of alligators," said Nancy.

"Bailing their skiff with a sieve," said Shelly, closing her eyes and lifting her face to the sun.

In late afternoon, Hack left the stickbird match and ambled over to join us. I could tell he'd been drinking. His eyes were dull and liquid, his balance precarious. Paul challenged him to a friendly round of skeet, and although the real contest was between Hack and Paul, we all joined in. Dudley released the targets as the others cried "Pull." Except for Mary Lou, who yelled "Sling it on!" or "Tarn that sucker a-loose!" When it was Paul's turn to shoot, he handed me the remote control.

Hack and Paul presented a remarkable contrast. Paul would take his stance, his gun shouldered. "Pull!" he called. I'd release the targets and watch him follow the birds as they left the houses, swinging smoothly through, breaking them neatly. When Hack shot, his stance was sloppy and unsteady, his marksmanship lethal. He had an almost comical lack of form. He would grunt to signal the release of the target, throw up his gun only after the birds had sailed onto the range. Elbows extended gracelessly, he fired without aiming as soon as the shotgun reached his shoulder, blasting targets out of the sky. I noticed he closed one eye when he fired, although Paul Dudley had instructed us to shoot with both eyes open. I asked him about it. "I got to close one eye to see which target to shoot," he grinned. "And which barrel to shoot it with."

"If he can shoot like that drunk," Nancy wondered aloud, "there's no telling what he could do sober."

"He can't hit the inside of a tobacco barn sober," Paul said. "I think he's scared of the noise."

"Yah hoo!" said Mary Lou, who was consistently breaking nearly every other clay pigeon. "This is as much fun as a gal can have with her clothes on." Her excitement was contagious. Some other members, including Country Trulane and Harry Defoe, drifted over, and Hack's marksmanship declined radically. In fact, he started missing targets regularly, receiving good natured teasing from us all. "I must be closing the wrong eye," he complained.

I introduced Country Trulane to Maloy, who remarked affably, "What's a city doctor doing out here in the sticks?"

"Shooting's my hobby," Dr. Trulane smiled. "Or one of them."

"What's the other ones?" asked Mary Lou, "besides clothes and cars." We'd shamelessly coveted Dr. Trulane's Jaguar when Shelly had parked the ambulance beside it. The ambulance and the XKE were conspicuous among the jeeps, Blazers, and pickup trucks.

"You like the Jag?" he smiled down at her.

"Course I do."

"You'll have to drive it sometime."

"You mean it?"

He didn't. "I also collect Native American artifacts." Trulane was anxious to change the subject. I guess he was afraid that Mary Lou would disappear over the horizon swirling red dust, peeking through the steering wheel.

"Arrowheads?" Maloy asked. Clearly Country Trulane wasn't the type to walk over newly plowed fields in muddy brogans, picking up flint.

"I have some points, yes, but I'm particularly proud of my ceremonial artifact collection." He winked at me. "I have one of the most select in the United States. Your brother-in-law will attest to my admiration of his snake-eye disk."

"Hack's got a big arrowhead collection," offered Mary Lou. "He keeps some of them at school for the kids. You ought to come out to the Junior High and see them sometime. I bet the kids never saw a Jaguar before. You can bring your arrowheads to show-and-tell."

"I'll have to do that," Country said with about as much enthusiasm for show-

151

and-tell as he had for turning Mary Lou loose in the XKE.

"Next week's O.K. with me."

"I'd have to check my calendar."

"Show-and-tell's next Thursday."

Trulane's mouth was fixed in a rictus grin. His eyes went flat.

"You done all right with that Ithaca, little lady," Harry Defoe interrupted. "Anybody shoots a gun that good ought to own it."

"I ain't got a gun," Mary Lou admitted.

My sister Nancy, the sociologist, pulled me aside. "Just take a look at *these* group dynamics," she whispered.

"Including you?" I whispered back, getting her point. Paul Dudley and Maloy were talking needs assessment and heath care grants. Hack was leaning on his shotgun, puffed up over the attention Mary Lou was shining on Country Trulane, the city doctor who flashed his bonded teeth and his XKE for us hayseeds. Shelly was chatting with a lanky Albert Defoe, the boy who'd outgrown the Ithaca, about his classes at Flint Junior College. Dan Defoe was trying to sell a shotgun, and Nancy was playing sociologist. A lot of electricity.

"What you want for it?" Hack pouted.

"Well, that's a special gun, my boy's first shotgun and all." Defoe scratched his whiskers. "I don't reckon I could sell her for less than a hundred dollars."

Albert overheard his father. "I cain't shoot it no more," he said, offering the obvious. The boy's left arm was longer than the Ithaca, butt to choke. His knuckles nearly drug the ground.

Harry's flinty eyes cut over to his son. "It's a fine little gun to train a youngun on," he said. "No offense, Miss Mary Lou."

"None taken," squeaked Mary Lou.

"What if I put up a hundred and fifty dollars against it and shoot you a round of stickbirds," Hack said, slurring his syllables. Whatever he'd been drinking was hitting him harder now, a delayed reaction. He was getting drunker by the minute. I wondered if he was too intoxicated to be handling firearms. If so, the only person around capable of taking his gun away from him was Shelly, who remained coolly polite, having suspended hostilities. Had she, for the collective good, decided to endure a separate peace?

"Wait a minute," snapped Mary Lou. "I can buy my own durn guns."

"Your big problem," Paul Dudley was telling Maloy, "is going to be Atlanta."

"Far out!" said Nancy.

"Well, lay down a hundred and fifty dollars then, Mary Lou," Hack said. "*That is* if Mr. Defoe finds them terms agreeable."

"Who'll sling?" Defoe wanted to know.

"Well, I ain't got $150 on me," cried Mary Lou. "I don't carry that kind of money on a date."

"We'll throw for one another," Hack told Defoe. "Best five birds."

"Loan me the money then," Mary Lou decided. "You can take fifty dollars a month out my pay if you lose."

"Fifty-five," said Hack. "To include interest on unsecured money."

"All right then, fifty-*five*," she said, stamping her foot, "but chivalry is dead as a hammer."

"You was wanting to buy your own damn gun two seconds ago," Hack said.

I was impressed. Hack stood to make fifteen dollars off Mary Lou just from losing a shooting match.

Defoe sent Alfred after the stickbird thrower, which was a hand-held Y-type sling spot-welded to a golf club. The extra length provided increased leverage which could hurl a clay target at what seemed supersonic speeds. Shooters had to fire quickly before the target sailed out of range.

"Anybody else want in?" Hack asked, looking dead at Country Trulane.

"Not me," Country said. "I'll shoot against you when you haven't been drinking."

Paul Dudley laughed. "There's a match that won't ever materialize."

"I think I'll shoot with them," Maloy said, "if Hack will give me back my twenty."

As Maloy stepped forward, Paul Dudley took his arm, winking and pulling him back.

Harry Defoe laid the Ithaca on the rough lumber trophy table, and Hack pulled out a roll of bills from the front pocket of his new Levis. He handed Maloy a twenty and wedged a wad of money under the stock.

"So that's what you had in them britches," Mary Lou said. "I thought you was just glad to see me when you come back from shooting them traps."

Hack grinned, stuffing the roll back into his pocket. "Step up here and take your first shot," he told Defoe. "I'll sling."

What happened next I have accepted as an optical illusion. Hack stepped forward with the stick in both hands, flexing his wrists like a golfer preparing to tee off and taking several deep breaths before spinning his body in a circle, like a discus thrower building momentum. Then faster than the eye could follow, the stick lashed, leaving Hack off balance, hopping on one foot. The clay target left the mouth of the thrower, seeming to pause in mid air, humming as it hovered with blurred edges before Defoe's astonished eyes. Then, before Defoe could shoulder his gun, the target with sudden incredible speed accelerated, quickly becoming a black spec on the horizon. By the time Defoe discharged his gun the target was out of range. "I wasn't ready," he said.

Defoe threw the next target, and Hack's firing pin clicked on an empty chamber. "I forgot to load up," he grinned. "I wasn't ready neither."

So they were one and one. The next target sailed straight away until the moment before Defoe fired, when it banked hard right and angled off unscathed. Defoe threw a "bird" with such force that it rattled with highspeed vibration and left him breathing deeply. Hack chipped the bird 50 yards out. "That was a lucky shot," raved Defoe.

Hack shrugged, throwing the next bird, which behaved like a rabbit on amphetamines. It flew close to the ground, riding updrafts and thermals at a fierce velocity that made it bounce and bound out to the horizon. Defoe missed again, cursing under his breath. Hack powdered Defoe's next two throws, taking an insurmountable lead.

"Double or nothing!" Defoe challenged. "You ain't walking away with my boy's first shotgun on a lucky chip!"

"O.K.," Hack said, limping over to the table for more shells. "Double or nothing on the next five."

"Oh no you ain't," screeched Mary Lou in a voice like a turntable arm dropped on a high speed record. "You ain't throwing away my new shotgun and my hard earned pay, and you too drunk to hit the ground with your durn hat!"

"You're wrong about that, Mary Lou," he said, taking off his Stetson and slapping it to the ground. His sun-burnished face met his pallid forehead at the sharp line his hat shaded. His hair was a disheveled gray and black.

"Let's go home," I said.

Hack hopped into the ambulance with surprising agility and immediately abandoned his alcoholic lisp. Maloy wanted to drive, so he and Shelly got into the cab.

"You ain't drunk!" Mary Lou scolded. "You played drunk to cheat them fellers shooting stickbird. And you call yourself a educator!"

"I played drunk to see if they'd try to cheat me. That double-or-nothing you locked the brakes on cost you a new dress."

"Oh, he's an educator all right," Nancy told Mary Lou. "He educated Harry Defoe, and he almost sent Jim Maloy to school."

"Well, at least I got me a new gun," said Mary Lou.

"That gun ain't worth twenty-five dollars," Hack said. "The hundred and fifty I put up was bait. I figured on driving off about sundown in Trulane's Jaguar. Maybe I'd won that Purdey."

"You was jealous," said Mary Lou proudly. "That's why you done that." She stood up and kissed him on the cheek. "And I'm right glad you ain't drunk. My daddy took drunk, and I can't stand to see it on a man."

I was, to borrow from the vernacular, happy as a buzzard on a dead hog. Paul Dudley had given me hope. And I was surrounded by friends and loved ones.

"Let's have supper next Thursday," Dr. Paul Dudley had said as we were leaving. He had flyers about rural health initiative programs circulating to my office. He said he'd look for a grant or two to help our indigent health care program. He even suggested joining the National Health Service Corps, which, he thought, would pay salaries for two more recruits.

The next morning I entered the following into my notebook:

--Sunday Oct. 9, 1983.

Shotgun gauges are determined by the number of lead balls the size of the muzzle necessary to make a pound. Thus a 20 gauge is twice as small as a 10 gauge, which would require one half the number of lead balls the diameter of the muzzle to equal 16 oz. This is true of all gauges except the .410 gauge, which is a caliber. (The muzzle of a .410 gauge is 410/1000 or 41/100 of an inch.) Shelly's "biological clock went off" at approximately four minutes after midnight (Oct. 10), sounding the alarm of conception, she said. O.S.

Chapter Thirty-Two

W hat do you think of these?" Mary Lou said in her scratchy, childlike voice. She'd walked brazenly to the chair where I studied her file, pulled open her blouse, and thrust her breasts into my face. "Well, what?" she insisted. With her blouse spread to her sides she looked like a proud bird drying its wings. Her breasts, though well formed, were the breasts of a much larger woman. They were close enough for me to nuzzle. I strained my neck backwards. She didn't want me to miss anything. I averted my eyes to her worried face. "Uh, nice breasts, Mary Lou." She'd made an appointment a couple of weeks after the picnic and had her records sent from Graves, her hometown and Country Trulane's.

"They too big or what?"

"Well, let's see," I said, "would you step back a little and give me some perspective." Actually Mary Lou had a voluptuous pair of breasts on an undersized body. "Have you noticed any lumps or tenderness?" I examined her breasts, which were firm and resilient with upright, healthy nipples.

She smiled, "They ain't been sore, and, no, there's no lumps. I was thinking more in line with one of those boob jobs, get them sized down a notch or two, you being a Hollywood doctor and all. I thought I might get them re-overhauled right here in town."

"You want a breast reduction?"

"Sure."

"Well, I'm not a Hollywood doctor. I went to Los Angeles for a few days to interview for a residency. I'm not a plastic surgeon, either. I'm an internist, and you might want to give the reduction idea some thought. Are you sure you want smaller breasts? Does Hack know you're thinking about a reduction?" Early May had reported that Hack and Mary Lou were already getting serious. He had taken her by the junkyard to meet his daddy, and they had visited his mother's grave. He was slated to meet her parents this weekend.

"Who cares a hairy rat's ass what he thinks." Her little forehead bunched into a frown. "If Hack Singletree wants to worry over somebody's titties, he can worry over his own. Course, he says he don't like the idea depriving younguns of a luxury before they're even born. I say they won't miss what they never had. He says just get one done and see how it goes, says I ought not to just jump whole hog into something like that."

"I don't think I'd recommend doing just one," I told her. "But I could refer you to a surgeon in Flint, and you could discuss it with him."

"Well, I don't like the idea of doing just one neither. I was just trying to show you what kind of thinking you're liable to hear from Hack Singletree on the subject. He also said my bubbies wasn't the only thing made me special, but they was two of the things that did." She thought for a moment; then she said, "You know, deep down in there, Hack Singletree is a rare gentleman." She was still airing her breasts when Early May stormed in to tell me that Frog Hullet was outside hooked up to a largemouth bass. Hack followed Early May in, looking for Mary Lou, stopping in mid-stride and cocking his head.

"Uh, tell Frog to come on back," I said. "Mary Lou, you can go ahead and rebutton your blouse. Hack, you aren't supposed to be back here."

"Looks like I came back here just in time to find my true love in a compromising situation and discover that my friend Mr. Hullet's done gone one-on-one with a largemouth bass," he grinned. "Now there's a sport!"

When Frog shuffled around the corner, it was all I could do to keep from laughing out loud. He was face-to-face, joined at the lips, with a three-pound bass, which he held tightly with both hands. Blood had drooled down his chin and dried. Tears had left trails through the grime. The bass was connected to Frog by a fishing lure, a Lucky 13, about the size of one of Bill Worthy's cheroots. Frog's nose was in the fish's mouth. It looked like he was blowing into the wrong end of a bugle. The fish was dead, apparently strangled, it's flared gills inlaid ruby red.

I sat Frog down in a chair while I fetched my wire cutters.

"Frog!" Hack hollered, bracing his hands on his knees, and leaning over to look in Frog's mouth. Since Frog was having trouble talking, Hack figured he couldn't hear either.

"Ut?"

"That's what I call giving the fish a even break. Damn if you ain't a thoroughbred!"

"How'd you do that?" Mary Lou asked, leisurely buttoning her blouse.

I clipped the shank of the treble hook embedded in Frog's lip to separate him from the bass, which I delivered to the sink. Frog could speak more clearly now, but his upper lip was puffed like a link of sausage, making his speech nasal. The hook jiggled as he talked.

"Well, how?" Mary Lou repeated.

"Thwallered the plug, and wooden come a-loose." Frog's face puckered and his eyes closed as he spoke.

"Well, how'd *he* get *you* is what I need to know." Her puzzled eyebrows bunched at the bridge of her nose.

"Got to shaking when I mit the line. Shook like a turpentine dog."

"You *bit* the line? Why didn't you cut him a-loose with your pocketknife?" Mary Lou wanted to know. She tucked in her blouse.

"'Sin my pocket. Muh hands was full," Frog mumbled, his face purpled with anger.

"Well, you shouldn't of bit it so close to the plug," she said. "Why'd you bite it so close?" She placed her fist on her hip.

"Let him be quiet, Mary Lou, until I can remove this hook." I examined the hook. One barb was buried from the inside in Frog's lip. I was going to have to push it through before I could cut off the barb and back it out."Close your eyes, Frog. These barbs may skip." Frog closed his eyes, shivering. Mary Lou and Hack cupped their eyes with their hands and watched on. I put on a pair of safety glasses. I clipped the other two flukes from the treble hook to safeguard against snagging him again. *Ping, ting.*

"New done, doc?"

"Not yet, I just started."

"Why'd he bite it so close?" she asked Hack.

"He must've reeled her up to the tip of his rod," Hack said.

"Is that what you done?" Mary Lou asked Frog.

"Don't make him talk, Mary Lou," I said. "Frog, I'm going to deaden this."

When Frog saw the novocaine needle, he shook his head and held me back. "Nat's migger than the hook," he mumbled.

"It's going to hurt when I pull it through," I assured him.

"Give him a shot of this," Hack said, producing a flask from his hip pocket. Frog turned up the flask, spilling the pungent liquid down his chin since he couldn't seal the neck of the bottle with his puffy upper lip. Hack's whiskey filled the office with fumes stronger than formaldehyde. Whiskey ran down Frog's chin, diluting the blood.

"I better have a shot too," Hack said. "It's hard to witness such misery."

"Doc?"

"No thanks."

He didn't offer whiskey to Mary Lou. Ladies didn't take whiskey straight from the bottle. Even Miss Ida, who could outdrink most men in the county, drank her undiluted spirits from a jelly glass or tumbler.

I pinched Frog's upper lip, grasping the shank with a clamp, but he kept rising out of the chair, following my hand and demonstrating the medical principle that when someone is pulling on a hook in your lip, you tend to come along. "Hold him," I ordered.

Hack squatted, wrapping his long arms around the back of Frog's chair and locking them around his chest. Frog kicked wildly, pivoting his head, twisting it, puffing his cheeks. "Watch his feet!" Hack warned.

"I ain't never seen such a baby," Mary Lou decided, stepping forward to grab a double handful of Frog's hair.

"Yahhhhh!" he yelled as I pushed the barb through. The tears squirted. His head vibrated violently, but Mary Lou and Hack held him fast. Mary Lou's own lips compressed, bloodless with determination.

"Youuuu!" Frog screamed as the dark point emerged like a thick whisker. I clipped the barb--*ting*--with the wire cutters and backed the hook out, leaving a tiny blue hole.

"You can let him go now, Hack," I said. "You too Mary Lou."

Mary Lou wiped her palms. Strands of oily hair were stuck to her fingers. She smelled her hands and made a face. "He's got Crisco in his head," she told me. "Did you hear me? He's got *Crisco* in his head!"

Hack grunted. His knees popped as he stood up. "Damn Frog," he said. "If a hooked fish pulled good as you, we'd never get one in the boat."

Chapter Thirty-Three

It became progressively clear that Dr. Dudley's prophesy was being fulfilled. Our reach exceeded our grasp. Grady's medical needs transcended our ability to fulfill them. With Flowers in detox and Hogue in the ground, the future of medicine in Grady weighed heavily on me and Maloy. Even with Trafford Memorial subsidizing our salaries, the office wasn't breaking even. Armed with quixotic enthusiasm and superior ivory tower medical training, we were locked in mortal combat with the cumulative pathology of 15,000 of our country's poorest souls. Against poverty, illiteracy, catastrophe, rural isolation, and destructive life styles, our battlements were overrun and the adversary windmill remained.

Jim and Nancy had been in town only a few weeks and already the waiting room was full and the waiting time for a new appointment was five days. At least I'd been getting some sleep every other night, but office finances had not improved much. We collected less than 50 cents on each dollar of charges we put on the books.

Nancy became our business manager, not a very smart move since her career purpose was to find services for the poor--she was finding medical services for the citizens of Grady, but *we* were becoming poor.

Even though Jim and I were on salary from the hospital, there was still a large loan to be paid off. The mystery around the trust sealing Hogue's office was being ostensibly explored by Morton Willetts, the hospital attorney, but little progress was being made, because Willetts was Wright's attorney too. The hospital desperately needed the office available to lease to potential family doctors or surgeons they were trying to recruit. Although the "head-hunting" firms were being paid $25,000, they informed us that without a rent-free office it would be difficult to compete with what other communities were offering. The hospital was strapped with decreased revenues and the cost of supporting our practice. The hospital census was rising, but still the red ink flowed. The loss of Hogue's surgeries and deliveries was devastating. Insurance companies are inclined to pay more for doing rather than thinking. Unfortunately, two internists think a lot more than they do.

Early May knew and loved everyone in Grady, and I'll be damned if she didn't rub off on Nancy. We became the safety net for the lost souls of society. Forty percent of Grady's population was below poverty, but sixty percent of our practice was. Nancy had stumbled across another Third World country and was trying to turn the office into a domestic branch of the Peace Corps. We did vocational counseling, stalled bank foreclosures, delayed discontinuation of utilities, enrolled people in Medicaid, and saved lives; but we had difficulty making our own payroll, and we missed installments on our loan. Grady's elite and insured preferred driving 25 miles to Flint to see *less* qualified internists and avoid sitting in the waiting room with the unwashed masses.

We yelled for reinforcements from the Public Health Service. Their brochures, at least, were encouraging. There were over 1,000 clinics in the poorest and most isolated locations of the country: Harlem; The Rosebud Indian Reservation in South Dakota; Mount Bayou, Mississippi. These clinics provided pharmacy, patient transportation, salaries for physicians, and even a method of recruiting obligated physicians through a new program called The National Health Service Corp. Nancy and Dr. Dudley wrote the regional office in Atlanta, requesting an application kit to convert our office into a Community Health Center. When our grant application kit arrived, we felt like we'd been delivered, that we'd died and gone to heaven. Miss Ivory Cleaver from the regional office would be coming down from Atlanta to assist us with the grant, and we anticipated her arrival as we would have awaited the angel of the annunciation. As soon as the date had been set for her visit, we contacted the people most concerned with the survival of the hospital and clinic and planned a premature supper celebration at Loonie Lake.

We fried catfish caught from Hack's set-hooks, trotlines, and fish baskets to christen our new "socialistic" venture. Melvin Dryden had welded a fish cooker fueled by propane. Miss Ida and Bill Worthy brought a five-gallon bucket of cole slaw, and we introduced the Maloys to hushpuppies, fried cornmeal cakes so named for their original use of pacifying hungry hounds at cookouts.

It was a festive, though exclusive, gathering of the folks most intimately involved in health care. The guest list included Margaret Holt; Early May; Denise; Buster Hogue; lab technician Billie Simmons; hospital administrator Andy Anderson; Ethel Hargrove's grandson James, the county's first black commissioner; Dr. Paul Dudley and Mrs. Rhodes, the public health nurse; Morton Willetts, chairman of the hospital authority *et all*; and Thomas Freelander, our master mason, who was accompanied by his grandson and Rooster Bootman, since Thomas was out past prison curfew.

Hack shook the fish in a brown bag with cornmeal and flower to bread them, then spit into the hot oil to test the temperature. The oil cracked and pinged metallically while five or six good-old-boys Maloy called *elders* nodded once in collective approbation. "Hit's hot, Hack," one of them pronounced.

Hack fried some sliced green tomatoes and breaded okra. He'd peeled sweet Vidalia onions and transected them into quarters three-fourths of the way through. Then he tossed them into the oil, where they foamed and fomented then blossomed like white flowers. Mary Lou served the onions on a platter like gardenias, their petals tinged brown around the edges. He fried the fish and then the hushpuppies, draining and keeping them warm in brown paper bags that absorbed the grease.

The fish fry was more or less without incident, not counting Shelly's accusation that Morton Willetts was involved in a conflict of interest by representing the Wrights and Trafford. She goaded him to his Cadillac with scalding censure. "You double-dealing, crawfishing son-of-a-bitch." I followed her to his car, putting my hand on her shoulder, trying to restrain her with gentle pressure.

Willetts entered the car and closed the door. Framed in the window, he held up his manicured hands calmly. "You'll see," he smiled ominously. "The practice of law is not the way you fashion it. It consists of deals, equivocations, and compromises. It's more concerned with pragmatism than justice. Come and speak with me again after you've finished with Vanderbilt and spent a few months in the trenches. You may even want to join my firm." This stopped Shelly cold. She'd spent a lot of time thinking about becoming an attorney, but she hadn't thought much about being one. If she returned to Grady without the money to open her own practice, she'd have to join an existing firm. She watched the solicitor's Cadillac drive cautiously away. Willetts was, for all practical purposes, the only game in town.

Hank grinned widely at Willetts' and Shelly's altercation, overjoyed that he, for once, was not the target of her wrath, but his attention lapsed when Lee Bob and Beulah arrived. He spilled hot grease, which ignited a paper tablecloth, causing temporary pandemonium. After a couple of drinks Shelly forgot Willetts. She and Mary Lou entertained with cheers and acrobatics. Mary Lou, perhaps overzealous to draw Hack's attentions from Beulah, did a series of cartwheels and roll overs, terminating in a back flip that exposed crimson bikini panties. The men began betting money on how many continuous combinations she could accomplish. Mary Lou's gyrations stretched, rolled, and compressed her D-cup breasts against centrifugal and gravitational forces inside her blouse. "Looks like two young coons fighting in a gunny sack," grinned Hack.

Hack's father, Elroy Singletree, in the rapture of his senility, stood enchanted by the pinwheel of the orbiting girl, mesmerized. Buzzard-like, his neck jutted perpendicular from his high, angular shoulders, and he wore a lopsided smile that seemed chopped into his deadpan face with an ax. Mr. Singletree was moved only by dismantling internal combustion engines and goggling Mary Lou, whose presence always called him from his uncharted fugue into some mindless joy. It was doubtful he recognized her from one meeting to the next. As was to be expected, Hack drank too much of Melvin's home brew, becoming goat-eyed, morose, and philosophical.

Shelly, Nancy, and Mary Lou had trouble concealing their instinctive feline distrust of Beulah, who flirted with Maloy shamelessly, raising his libido, Hack's hackles, and my secret chagrin. Although I didn't want to be attracted to Beulah, I couldn't help being drawn to the incredible magnetism she radiated like phermomes. Even Nancy, who was accustomed to Maloy's naturally outgoing and flirtatious manner, was visibly irritated, but Maloy, always able to defuse potentially explosive situations, broke away from Beulah and made a beeline to Hack, offering to help with the fish. Beulah's seductive eyes followed Maloy to the fish cooker. "That's some gal," Maloy told Hack, "but she's got the hots for you and you alone. Look at the way she's eyeballing you right now."

After supper we had a discussion of the hopeful possibility of our clinic's conversion to a Community Health Center. Most present were optimistic, a notable exception being Beulah and Lee Bob Parker, who said the scheme was an invitation to socialized medicine. "What's wrong with that?" Margaret Holt wanted to know.

"You folks ought to be tired of the government coming down here with one program or the other screwing things up and calling it the common good . . ." Lee Bob Parker began. He was casually dressed in a navy Polo shirt and penny loafers.

"Like the *abolitionists*?" Margaret demanded.

Jim Maloy, the diplomat, was on his feet. "Excuse me, folks, but I'm afraid if we start our discussion with the War of the Confederate Secession, we might yaw a bit afield before we arrive at the point of our discussion. We are here," he said, "to celebrate the possibility of rescuing Grady's health care program with a federal grant."

My brother-in-law was slick. How easily and naturally he gauged people and situations, intuitively knowing that the *Civil* War was an improper appellation for a subject that was still a Southern bone of contention after more than a century.

When I first arrived at Grady, I'd been amused by the lingering sensitivity to antebellum issues. I asked Hack about it, and he'd replied with a wink, "We're still occupied by the enemy down here--U.S. military bases, reconstructionists, carpetbaggers, industrialists, hot-shot doctors--we're still under siege, that's why. But I never thought I'd hear an *Irish*man complain about a dispute that's gone on a mere hundred years. At least we quit shooting minnie balls at you boys."

Chapter Thirty-Four

Ivory Cleaver was a porcine female in her early thirties, ten pounds over the maximum capacity of her white knit dress, which stretched over the lower third of an ample white bosom. Her turned-up nose made me afraid I'd get an unwanted peek at her brains. I met her at the Flint airport and set out in the Falcon for Lake Loonie, where we were to join Shelly, Nancy, and Maloy. Ivory taught me what it meant to be imprisoned by bureaucracy. I learned to sympathize with Southerners' typical suspicion of outsiders, of bureaucrats empowered by distant imperial governments--emissaries who descend to impoverished colonies rendering difficult situations hopeless with memorized regulations.

Miss Cleaver's victims were bound in webs of endless red tape. "I don't want to put no sand in your Vaseline," Hack warned when I first told him a bureaucrat was scheduled to come, "but the most obvious lies in America today are: 'Your check's in the mail'; 'I'll still respect you in the morning'; and 'I'm from the gov'ment, I'm here to help you.'"

"Welcome, Miss Cleaver," I said. "We're honored you agreed to come down to help us with the rather, uh, desperate medical needs we face at Grady."

"Oh, I'm not here to help you," she began. "You'll have to *prove* your needs are indeed desperate. I'm here to tell you that you must fill out a 300-page grant and to advise you that you will be in stiff competition with many larger and better organized communities." She applied vermilion lipstick in the rear view mirror as we started back to Grady. The conversation went downhill for the next eight hours.

When we got to my house, it didn't take long for my group to discover that getting help from Miss Cleaver was going to be like squeezing sweat from a rock. But Nancy was used to advocating the social needs of the downtrodden. "Surely, Ms. Cleaver," she began, "you know we're not asking for special favors. We realize that Public Health Grants follow strict criteria for eligibility and accountability. But my husband and brother genuinely want to make a difference here in Grady."

"Your sacrifices are, um, noteworthy," Ivory Cleaver said adjusting her dress, "but the 330 Section of the Public Health Service Act specifically states that the Community Health Center must be owned and directed by a 51% majority *consumer* board of directors. We are not in the business of bailing out physicians who are unable to make a go of it in their private practice."

Shelly looked ready to check out the roots of Ivory's lacquered eggplant hair when Maloy interceded. "We're ready to make sacrifices necessary to improve health care in Grady. If we turn the clinic over to the community and establish a proper governing board, then what would it take to get the grant funds?"

Miss Cleaver handed over 42 pages of Program Expectations; 136 pages of the *Primary Care Effectiveness Review*; a 200 page manual, *The Bureau of Common Reporting Requirements*; and there were others, to the tune of 1,000 pages of rules, regulations, and directions for the grant application. "You have until December 1--45 days--to fill out the application, which must strictly adhere to the guidelines contained within the Grant Application Kit. Do you have any questions?"

We realized the task was impossible, but we also knew that this grant was the only salvation for medical care in Grady. It was obvious that Miss Cleaver didn't give a sailing shit if we got the grant or not. Months of frustration, exhaustion, and dashed hopes became personified by a saucy bureaucrat in a stressed knit dress. Sick patients against paperwork.

Shelly, understanding that our survival boiled down to one more grant application Ivory Cleaver would have to evaluate, was first to anger. She compared Miss Cleaver's usefulness to that of *tits on a boar hog*, reminding her that she was a civil servant whose salary was paid by taxes. Shelly demanded the name of her supervisor, whom she wanted to contact to determine why uncooperative Miss Cleaver, who was so obviously insensitive to the needs of her constituency, was allowed to wiggle and strut so insolently with the assumed power of a federal agency. "These doctors--Stone and Maloy--don't need Grady," Shelly continued. "Grady needs them! This community deserves that grant, and you know it. You can bet your dimpled ass your supervisor's going to know it too."

Miss Cleaver smiled tightly. "As an official of the Public Health Service, my duty is to uphold the rules and regulations of the Public Health Services Act," she recited. "It is your job and your responsibility to submit your application; we will judge it on the technical merits contained within."

Maloy's Irish was up. His jugular veins swelled with rage and his eyes bulged from intracranial tumescence caused by an increase of hydraulic pressure. I was worried that he'd rupture a blood vessel. That or cheerfully murder Miss Ivory Cleaver where she stood in overleaven red pumps. "I'll see to it that you get to the airport," I offered quickly. I wasn't in any way inclined to spend what was left of the day driving her. Nancy called Melvin Dryden. It took every penny the four of us could scrape together to send Miss Cleaver to the airport, but it was worth it--the best money we'd ever spent. I ushered her quickly into the yard to wait for Melvin, leaving Maloy and Shelly, their foreheads nearly touching, muttering murderous obscenities. Their common adversary gone, I was afraid they'd turn on each other. "Get Maloy a drink," I told my sister. "There's medicinal moonshine in the cabinet over the stove."

Round one went to the bureaucrats. And to Melvin Dryden, who got paid wrecker service fees for speeding her to Flint.

Chapter Thirty-Five

W e worked harder on the grant than we'd ever worked on anything before, harder than we had worked in med school and college. It was a group effort, all-nighters with pizzas and gallon jugs of Chianti wine imported from Flint. Denise did the typing, Nancy and Shelly wrote and revised. They provided the rhetoric, diction, and syntax, while Maloy and I organized, researched information, and gathered data. Getting together a community board was easily accomplished. Commissioner Worthy's wife, Miss Ida, served as chairman. Mr. Anderson; Margaret Holt; one of Miss Ethel's granddaughters, Tessie Mae Miller; and the public health nurse, Mrs. Rhodes served on the board. Dr. Paul Dudley got up the needs assessment, a document that described the medical, geographic, and social realities of the community to be served. Nancy investigated the structure of the regional office in Atlanta and got the name of the Primary Care section Chief, who happened to be an old friend of Nancy's Health Policy instructor at Stanford. Small World. No, small network.

"Jessanne Lockwood is, now hear this," Nancy said, hanging up the telephone, "a *caring*, quality health administrator and a supervisor of our beloved Ivory Cleaver."

Jim Maloy had friends everywhere, too. One of them, Bernie Poulos, did *locum tenens* work out of Atlanta. He agreed to cover our practice as we undertook the second Battle of Atlanta.

Dr. J. Puckett Middlebrooks, an OBGYN with a four-seated Cessna, flew the Maloys and me from Flint to the Atlanta Airport. The good natured Middlebrooks, who'd helped us with several tough deliveries, was blessed or cursed with the physiognomy of perpetual youth. "Puck" looked adolescent and often acted so. Early in his career, he'd tended an emergency in the delivery room only to be ordered out by the patient. "Get that goddamn kid outa here!" the husky housewife had cried when Puck's childish face appeared between her knees. He left and returned, wearing a beanie with a plastic propeller. "You've had Lamaze," he said. "Just huff till you see this propeller spin, and we'll make a mother out of you."

The first cold snap had begun to burnish the hardwoods of the Piedmont Plateau red and gold. From the air, I found myself proudly pointing out to Jim and Nancy another aspect of Georgia's multi-faced natural beauty as though it were my homeland. Ironically, most of my knowledge of Georgia's geography, from the barrier islands and glens of the Atlantic coast to the rugged mountains of Appalachia, I had learned by way of slide presentations and books Miss

Tappie Handson had made available at the library. I was buried too deep in Georgia to get an overview.

We landed at the Atlanta airport, where we rented a Volkswagen sedan and drove beneath the gold domed Capitol and the skyline of chrome and smoky glass to the office of Jessanne Lockwood. As we walked down Peachtree, Maloy was amazed by the number of beautiful women tending shops, waiting for cabs, or walking the sidewalks in the brisk autumn air. "They actually look you in the eye and smile," he marveled. "What kind of a city is this?"

Puck grinned, informing us he'd planned to team up with an old college pal, Canterbury Pace Davison. They'd be at the Piedmont Driving Club for drinks and dinner if we needed to get in touch. If not, we could meet him back at the hanger at *dark thirty*.

"*College* Pal?" Nancy teased. "How could you have a college pal? You don't look old enough to have gone to college."

Maloy's first question for Mrs. Lockwood was, "Does Miss Cleaver have to be our project officer?" The prospect of dealing with an actual human being instead of a bureaucrat automaton put us at ease.

"Not unless you are planning a hazardous landfill," answered the immaculately dressed, well-mannered woman with a Mississippi Delta drawl. She insisted we call her Jessanne. "I laterally transferred Miss Cleaver to the Nuclear Regulatory Commission on the 7th floor," she said, winning our hearts. "By the way, Mrs. Maloy, I appreciate your candor concerning Ivory's attitude. The recent Carter administration doubled the funding in our 330 section, and PHS personnel policy forced us to base the massive hiring that followed on civil service seniority. Miss Cleaver was an IRS secretary three months ago, so her conduct is understandable, if inexcusable."

"I'll sleep better with Ivory in toxic wastes," said Maloy.

"Let me give you my spiel," said Jessanne Lockwood, "with just a touch of personal note, which I hope you'll find encouraging: My father was the only family doctor for 6,000 people in an impoverished area in the Delta. I remember the poverty, the shortage of funds for tests and medications, the magnitude of health problems. I think I know what you're up against in Grady."

We encountered one more obstacle. Somebody else had applied for the grant within a 30-mile area, in south Flint. If we would agree to a merger, we'd get preference and treble our point total in the review process. In other words, the merger would put our grant in the bag. "What the hell," grinned Maloy. "We might as well go big time, open a nationwide chain like Col. Sanders."

We'd instantly grow from a two-man rural clinic to a network of health facilities, which was just about the best wad of red tape we could find. On Jessanne's's recommendation, former civil rights activist Wade Perdew wrote the consolidation grant. He'd never heard of Grady but had been jailed in Flint, which he remembered more fondly than Selma, Alabama, where he was bitten by a German police dog.

Within two weeks Wade would transform two orange crates of paper and data into a 368 page grant that would bring us $395,000. We'd be able to help patients pay for drugs, and we'd be able to have a social worker and health educator attached to the clinic. But the greatest benefit was that Maloy and I would be able to join The Public Health Service and have them pick up our salaries. We'd also receive an invitation to the National Health Service Corp's version of "Supermarket Sweep," where we could recruit obligated physicians who had borrowed federal money for med school. The National Service Corps had become the most successful program for distributing quality physicians to underserved communities.

"Socialized medicine!" screamed Puck Middlebrooks over the drone of his Cessna. "I've become a shuttle for Boskies, Marxists, and Yankee carpetbaggers!" He put the airplane into a series of congratulatory loops and aerial acrobatics. I turned green, Maloy crossed himself, and Nancy threw up into a wax-coated bag. Never again, we swore, would we fly with Dr. Middlebrooks, especially after one of his inspiring sessions at the Piedmont Driving Club with Canterbury Pace Davison.

Chapter Thirty-Six

From my office I called Dr. A. Hamilton "Country" Trulane to ask him to screen some of my patients with eye problems. He accepted too readily. It wasn't like Trulane to work for nothing, although God knows he could afford to.

"Pull them in Wednesday week?" he said. "I'll come over Wednesday morning and we'll shoot Tailfeathers in the afternoon."

"I can do that," I said. "I've got some questions to ask you about the snake-eye disk. I may let you take it home for a few days to study."

"Sure, but promise me you'll hang on to it until then."

I didn't think Dr. Trulane was going to be able to wait until Wednesday week to talk about the disk, and I was right. In fact, Early May told me he was waiting to see me within 45 minutes from the time I hung up the phone. "Well, let's see it," he grumbled as though inconvenienced by his drive over from Flint. I asked him why this disk was different from Mr. Mack's disk in the library. He didn't seem surprised that the workmanship was more crudely executed than on the Jones' disk.

"It's stylistically the same," he said, running his finger reverently over the eye that was etched into the open palm at the center of the disk. "Usually, the eye is associated with the sun, and the hand represents a benediction, perhaps from the heavens. The snakes are the lords of the underworld, representing the potent blessings of the earth. Due to its lack of patina, I don't think this individual piece is very old, certainly no more than a couple hundred years, but the tradition could be thousands of years old. It doesn't make any difference *when* the individual artist lived. The creation of the disk is a timeless act, which has nothing to do with the individual artist."

Dr. Trulane held the disk as though it were made of the finest, most fragile Chinese porcelain. The way its presence moved him was almost absurd, a fetish.

"What do you mean it doesn't have anything to do with the artist?" I got a Coca-Cola from the drug cooler and offered one to Dr. Trulane, who shook his head.

"It's only in recent times that the individuality of the artist has been considered important. I mean, if you buy a Picasso, you want it signed. You appreciate Picasso for his singularity, his uniqueness, but the value of ancient art is diminished by any traces of the artist, whose vision should be uniform with that of his predecessors' and pure to the extent that it is untainted by the hands that create it." What Trulane was saying sounded consistent with Hack's dictum, "The ancient artist is a vehicle of that pure and perfect vision that isn't altered by individual artists."

"Do you mean that the creator of the disk sort of goes into a trance and stamps out icons in perfect accord with some archetypal image?"

"Well archetypal's a good word. The serpent-eye motif is a common combination that predates Roman times, in fact all of the elements of the disk carry us back to pre-historic old world beginnings, but this artist was trained from childhood in a timeless tradition passed down from generation to generation for the purpose of creating one icon only or a few at most of the same basic subject."

"Could the disk in the library and this disk have been done by the same artist?"

Dr. Trulane smiled enigmatically. "Well, it's possible, but not likely. Even if both disks were made in this area, the same motif could've been reproduced for several centuries. Add to that the possibility that the disks could have been traded by Indians traveling through this area from somewhere else, although I don't think so. It's unlikely that Indians would trade sacred artifacts, which is what the disks seem to be."

"What if the artist lost his eyesight between making the disk in the library and this one?" I'm not sure what I wanted Trulane to say, but it's possible I was trying to lead him to a collaboration I'd promised Hack I wouldn't divulge.

"Sure." Trulane's smile drifted to one side of his mouth. "Or he could have contracted Parkinson's disease. Or crawled around a jug of firewater. Or been scared witless by a saber-tooth tiger."

Seeing Dr. Trulane's Jaguar in my office parking lot, Hack must have rushed home for his own disk and returned. He barged in with it wrapped in the chamois. "I got a deal for you," he told Country Trulane without even a preliminary hello.

"Let's hear it," said the ophthalmologist.

Basically Hack's deal was that he would bet his disk against a free cataract operation for Potter Fish Kinnard in a stickbird contest the following Wednesday. Hack refused to swap the disk outright for the services because that was too much like selling the icon, which would bring on considerable bad medicine. Gambling for it was acceptable because it would encourage participation of the Great Spirit, who could smile or frown upon the fortune of the participants. Country Trulane was astounded to discover that three snake-eye disks existed in Grady County. Being in the presence of two of them seemed to rattle him.

"What's in this for you?" he wanted to know.

"That's my business," Hack squinted. "We got a bet or not?"

"O.K.," agreed Trulane, "Who'll throw?"

"Anybody you say. What about Dr. Paul Dudley? He's at Tailfeathers every

Wednesday."

"Done," said Country Trulane. "I'll call him."

"What *is* in it for you?" I asked Hack after Trulane had left, "and what's all the bullshit about the Great Spirit smiling down on the participants."

"That weren't bullshit," Hack grinned, "but I sure am proud to see you're finally learning how to talk. The Great Spirit has already smiled down on my cloven ass, making me a better shot than Trulane and sending me a sucker who can knock the scales off the Chief's eyesight." He paused to hitch his low-riding khakis beneath his overleaven belly. "Just like the Great Spirit smiled on the Chief by sending him a sucker to cure his dropsy."

"Why didn't we just ask Trulane to take the operation as a charity case? And why are you so interested in taking Trulane on at stickbirds."

"Point one: he's a Wright. He's Karl's sister's son, so he ain't going to do it without getting something back. Point two: I don't want to owe the son-of-a-bitch nothing, and the Chief don't neither. Point three: is I'm beholding to the Chief just like he's beholding to you. We get the cataracts shucked off his eyes, everybody's got a clean slate."

"Why are you beholding to Fish Kinnard?"

"Why he's the one taught me to shoot."

Chapter Thirty-Seven

The following Wednesday Country Trulane came to the clinic like he'd promised. I'd scheduled 45 patients with serious eye problems who were not being seen by an ophthalmologist. Trulane expected four or five. "I don't see how this is possible," he said. "I have the largest ophthalmologic surgical practice in the Southeast. I did over 600 lens implants last year. Why haven't I seen some of these people?"

"I don't mean to be critical, but I've found it practically impossible to get Medicaid *or* indigent patients in to see you. My medicare and 100% insured patients are worked into your system within a week."

"I was told we're seeing everybody who comes to us."

"Who told you that?"

"Karl Wright handles the business end. He did, but I'll check on it anyway when I get back to the Flint office."

Dr. Trulane set up his slit lamp. He wanted to do visual fields testing and tonometry as well as direct fundoscopic examinations and tests for visual acuity. His first patient was Madeiline Hunter, a 45-year-old insulin dependent diabetic who was on 45 units of NPH insulin a day. Madeiline's husband died two years before. Her vision had degenerated to the point she couldn't care for herself or her three children.

Trulane dilated her eyes, observed her, then motioned me to follow him into the adjoining room. "Christ, Stone, this woman has a detached retina. She should've had laser photocoagulation two or three years ago. She'll be blind in six months."

"I treated her for diabetic ketoacidosis. When I saw her eye grounds, I referred her. She sat in your waiting room four hours, was told you had an emergency and that she'd be called back for an appointment. She didn't hear from your office, so she called three times asking for an appointment. She could go to the medical college, but that's three or four hours from here and she can't drive. She's decided if she can't get treated here, she'll have to 'leave it up to the Lord.'"

Trulane shook his head. "I'll post her for a vitrectomy next week and see if I can do something to stabilize her vision."

His next patient was a sixty-two-year-old woman with substantial glaucoma. Then he saw Donnie Jacobs, a sixteen-year-old who'd developed a conjunctivitis that really worried me. "I did a fluorescein stain that had a dendritic pattern that could have been herpes," I told Trulane. "I called the ER at Putnam, who referred him to Southern Vision. The ER M.D. said to try to get the ophthalmologist to see him as an outpatient. I called your office and was told that you weren't taking any new patients--that the only way I could get Donnie seen was through the ER. His family lives out in the sticks. They gave up trying to get help, and when they brought him back to me in six months, he had what appeared to be a scarred cornea."

"Donnie," Trulane said, "I know you can't see very well, but we can help you. I'm going to personally arrange a cornea transplant just as soon as we can find a matching cornea."

"Excuse us, Donnie," I said. I pulled Trulane out into the hall. "Dr. Trulane, you'd better know this kid's parents are uninsured, like about half of the patients in my practice. Don't get his hopes up if we can't follow through."

"Let me worry about this one," Trulane smiled. "That kid can't shoot dove or see the girls in 3-D if we don't get him a new cornea. What kind of life can he have unable to see girls in the round? I've got some Lions Club connections. We should be able to get funding for the transplant, and I'll donate my services."

Early May came back. "Singletree's got a man out there you might want to see so you can get them on out of here."

"What's that smell?" asked Country Trulane. "You got a campfire in there?" By the smell of wood smoke and garlic, I knew that Hack had managed to extract Fish Kinnard from the Swamp of Toa.

Kinnard was sixty pounds lighter. The hatchet of his nose seemed even larger than it had when I'd spent the night at his cabin. His leathery cheeks, the color and texture of dried persimmons, had deep stork tracks from the corners of his eyes to his ears. His neck was crimped like oak bark. With his fluids drained, he'd shrunk inside his skin.

Hack led him in, helped him into a chair, and acted as his spokesman. "Because Dr. Otis Stone has done Mr. Fish Kinnard a great service," Hack translated, "Mr. Kinnard has accepted the white doctor's invitation to visit him in this office. He is prepared to stay two days at the house of his friend Elroy Singletree, so that the eye doctor can remove the blindness."

"They're ripe," Trulane said of the cataracts. "See the white reflection caused by the smoky haze on the cornea? There's no red reflex. Notice how dead eyes look when you can't see into the retina." He turned to Hack. "You're pretty sure about winning our bet," he observed.

Hack raised his index finger to his lips and motioned me and Country Trulane into the next room. He leaned over and scrutinized Trulane with his right eye while he closed the other by torquing the entire left side of his face into a wad. This was to show that he had a serious proposition. "Now, I'm still prepared to go best out of three for my disk," he said. "But me and the doc here's got two disks. If it's O.K. with the doc, we'll wager them both. If I win, we keep both disks and you fix up the Chief. If I lose, you keep both disks and fix up the Chief too. This way the Chief gets his operation either way and we avoid pissing off the Great Spirit by swapping out directly."

Trulane's eyes glazed over. He had been trying all of his adult life to acquire a snake-eye disk. Now he had a clear shot at two.

"I'll go along," I agreed. "Easy come, easy go."

"The Chief says you got to do it tonight or tomorrow morning, so he can get his sight back and go on home. He don't want to get contaminated by staying too long in town."

I smiled, but the sobering fact crossed my mind that before the coming of the white man, Native Americans were practically free of contagious diseases. Influenza, smallpox, and the common cold brought by the Spaniards killed them by the thousands.

"I've got a full schedule tomorrow," said Trulane, "but I guess I could get some equipment sent over to Trafford and do it before seven in the morning if Trafford will grant me temporary privileges, but Mr. Kinnard needs both eyes done."

"So do them both," Hack said. "It don't matter to the Chief. I know I ain't going to be able to get him back to town again until the doc saves his life again. He's blind now. He don't care if there's one bandage on his eyes or two by tomorrow."

"Can't you operate here at the office?" I wondered.

"I'd rather be in the Trafford OR, and there's one more problem. By the time I see all the patients Dr. Stone has lined up for me today, it may be dark."

"That don't matter. You're obliged to fix the Chief's eyes win or lose. We can shoot the match later, or if you want to, we can shoot under lights. There's floodlights at Tailfeathers, ain't there? It don't make a dime's worth of difference to me when we shoot or where."

I knew they'd shoot as soon as Trulane could finish examining my patients. He was obsessed with the prize, and he'd be too excited to postpone the match. He must have also considered a nighttime match as an advantage. Hack couldn't possibly have gained any experience shooting under lights. He didn't believe in night hunting, which was about the only illegal activity he disapproved of besides selling drugs in the schoolyard. Trulane was banking on Hack's pupils being dilated by alcohol. He figured Hack would be sloshed by nightfall, as usual. "I'll see you in the morning, Mr. Kinnard," he said as we returned from our conference to the room where Kinnard sat like chiseled stone. He gazed blindly at our voices, nodding once before Hack led him away.

Trulane was amazed to see so many patients who had fallen through the hole in the system. "You told me you had some tough cases," he admitted, "but frankly I'm shocked by the severity of the ophthalmologic pathology you've had to manage. I thought you'd have a few people who needed refraction to get fitted for glasses. Your patients are going blind for lack of attention."

When we finished seeing all 45 patients, he still found it incomprehensible that these people weren't getting cared for. He didn't know about them because his front office wasn't telling him. Why should they? On a busy day, Trulane could do ten cataract operations and bring in $20,000 for himself and $40,000 for Southern Vision. Country Trulane didn't lack humanity, but the system did. Karl Wright's business manager saw only the bottom line, which is what Southern Vision was all about.

"Will you come back to Grady sometime?" I smiled, "or have I run you off permanently."

"I think so," Trulane said seriously. "Something's wrong with this. A deal's a deal, but why isn't that Indian on Medicare?"

"He's never had a paycheck, never paid a cent into Social Security. He's not registered for any type of benefits."

"How does somebody like that get by?" Trulane mused. On a slow day Country probably had to eke by on a grand or two.

"He can't without his eyesight, but listen, you should be honored. This trip to town was probably his first visit to a trained physician other than a root doctor. He has chronic hypertension and congestive cardiomyopathy. I had to spend the night out in the swamp with him to give him IV Lasix and Digoxin. Hack takes blood pressure medication out to him every three months. The only reason he came to town today is because he can't refuse me. I saved his life."

"That's impressive, but how does this character eat? What does he do for money?"

"He farms Mulgrove Ridge some. Hunts, fishes, traps, barters with his neighbors, makes a little shine, keeps some goats and chickens. He's an extreme case, but you'd be surprised at how many people there are in this county in similar circumstances, people who have absolutely no prospects of health care."

"Well, I grew up in this area, but the amount of untreated pathology around here is shocking even to me."

Chapter Thirty-Eight

D r. Paul Dudley let the cat out of the bag that Dr. Country Trulane had been honing his impressive skills, practicing stickbirds at the Tailfeathers Skeet and Trap Club every night since Hack challenged him. Of course, Hack didn't need to practice at Tailfeathers. This was December, the tail end of hunting season. Hack hunted game birds regularly--the dove, the swamp quail, the woodcock, the snipe, the wood ducks in and on the fringes of the Swamp of Toa, where birds flew wildly through dense cover. Hack had been in continuous practice, more or less, since he was nine years old.

Elroy Singletree and Fish Kinnard were left in the care of Mary Lou with my strict instructions that the old men not drink stump or red whiskey. I asked Hack to stay sober too, in order not to stack the odds against the Great Spirit's benevolent patronage. When he arrived, he smelled like a pickled pig's foot but was walking straight enough. He'd brought his rattlesnake disk and I'd brought mine. We laid them side-by-side on the rough-hewn boards of the trophy table while Paul Dudley articulated the rules, which were simple and straightforward.

Tossing a coin to determine who was to shoot first, the marksmen took turns shooting with their own guns and #9 shot. Targets were declared hit when they broke into at least two visible pieces. The winner was to be the first shooter to gain a two-point advantage.

It was a slow, dull, and exhausting match. Trulane, having changed in my office, wore an expensive leather shooting jacket and kid gloves. He wore a bright red ascot and amber shooting glasses. He stepped to the line shouldering his hand-engraved Purdey, breaking his birds in perfect form of the English landed gentry he had married into.

Hack, in rude contrast, wore brogans and overalls, his everpresent Stetson cocked rakishly to one side. He carried his shotgun shells in a nail pouch that advertised Gary Weed's Hardware and hung like a baggy sporran under his belly. He followed Trulane, spitting tobacco juice from a wad of Levi Garrett that distorted his jaw. He stepped forward, calling for the bird with a rude grunt, throwing up with elbows high and breaking targets with his disreputable pump-action shotgun, silvered with wear and bound at the cracked stock with friction tape.

In the chilly December evening, Paul Dudley huffed vapor and broke into a sweat. The shooters broke 100 targets without any indication that they would ever miss one. The north wind resumed soon after dusk, causing the birds to fly erratically, but still the shooters hit consistently. Paul rested to regain control, but the targets still flew more and more awry. Trulane was a graceful, schooled, and disciplined skeet and trap marksman, but Hack was an instinctive and deadly meat hunter, who'd learned at an early age to bag wild birds from thickets, hedge rows, canebrakes, and briars. He was a snap shot, an instinct shooter, whom the unexpected did not disadvantage.

I felt sorry for Country Trulane even though my wager was with the opposition. The worse the conditions became, the more obvious it became that Hack would win. Although neither man had missed, Trulane was breaking targets while Hack powdered them.

The first target Trulane missed would have been called foul on any range but this one. The clay disk stuck in the mouth of the thrower, becoming airborne late in the swing so that it wobbled off at a harsh right angle to the shooter, whose firearm was shouldered for a 12 o'clock target. Trulane's second miss was a bird slung low so that it dipped and bounced along in the gusty ground wind. Hack shattered such targets without a second thought, since he never anticipated the direction of any target. He threw up his gun only after he'd seen the target broken in his mind. If Paul had managed to throw a clay pigeon behind the shooters, it wouldn't have made any difference to Hack.

When the contest was finally over, Paul Dudley was stumbling tired. I couldn't have relieved him even if I'd known how because I wasn't a disinterested party. Trulane had seen Hack throw stickbirds and refused to accept the conditions that the shooters throw for each other, but after his second miss he proved to be a good loser. He shook Hack's reluctant hand. "See you first thing in the morning for the Indian's cataracts," he said. He walked over to the rattlesnake disks, took a longing last look. I could tell he was brokenhearted, devastated. The snake-eye disks were one of the few things he'd ever wanted that he couldn't have. "Nice shooting, Hack," he said again. "I'll have to get you to give me some lessons."

"I thought I just did," Hack mumbled, spitting a caramel stream of tobacco.

Early the next morning I observed Kinnard's cataract removal and lens implant. The tall Indian, his cloudy eyes held open and wide by the retractors, looked like a strange night bird. With the dexterity he was famous for, Trulane made a small incision on the edge of Kinnard's cornea, removed and replaced the lens, and sutured the original incision with thread smaller than a human hair. When he'd finished both eyes, he bandaged them and told us to meet him in my office the next morning.

Hack and I led the old Indian back to his truck. "I guess you're welcome to stay one more night, Chief," Hack said, "but after tomorrow you got to go back to the Toa. I'm scared if you stay in Grady too long, you and the old man'll get to scalping the Sunday school teachers and Colonial Dames."

The following morning, when Dr. Trulane returned to Grady and unwound the bandages from the old Indian's eyes, I had trouble repressing my excitement. Kinnard sat proud and straight in his chair until the patches were taken from his eyes--eyes which were now clear and black. He blinked. Then he blinked again, and his jaw dropped. He looked around the room, until his dumbfounded gaze fell on Hack. "Hack!" he screamed. "Hack!"

"I'm right over here, Chief."

Kinnard's watering eyes widened with recognition. "Hot damn," he said, grinning a formless smile that nearly touched his nose to his chin. "I'd fergot what a ugly sumbitch you was." He stared at Dr. Trulane. He looked at me. Then he looked at the backs of his hands, and he turned again to Country Trulane. "You the one that fixed my eyes?" he asked without a trace of gentleness or appreciation.

Trulane nodded.

"I'm right obliged," said Kinnard.

Chapter Thirty-Nine

I've killed all of my friends!" whispered a hysterical Mrs. Van Schench into the telephone, "and a good number of Senator Richardson's constituents."

"How?" I managed. I was struggling out of deep, much coveted sleep. Shelly bolted up to one elbow, "I've got to go home," she declared without waking up. I turned on the bedside lamp and glanced at my watch. It was only 10 p.m.

"How'd you kill them, Mrs. Van Schench?"

"My shrimp mousse!" she hissed. "I've poisoned everybody, including Mildred Hesse." Mildred Hesse was the president of the Colonial Dames. "Oh, and my husband," she added. "Oh my God, and I've even killed Senator Richardson."

"Why are you whispering? Where are the people you've poisoned?"

"They're having dessert, and I don't want them to hear me," she whispered. "Oh, this just spoils everything. You're just going to have to rush right over here and pump out everybody's stomach."

"How do you know you poisoned them?" I yawned.

"Miss Penny died in the kitchen. She threw up . . . *blood*!"

"Miss Penny?"

"My miniature poodle!" she whispered conspiratorially. Then I *knew* I was dreaming. "Doctor, you are wasting precious time. Everybody will start dropping dead at any moment."

"What time is it?" mumbled Shelly in her sleep.

"How many people are there? How many people have you poisoned?"

Mrs. Van Schench was from the old order of Southern aristocracy, educated at exclusive women's colleges where they learned to arrange flowers and stick toothpicks in olives. "Well, let's see," she said. "Fifteen couples were on the guest list, but some regretted."

"I'll bet!"

"No, I'm mean they sent word that they were predisposed and unable to attend."

"You've poisoned thirty people? What with?"

"I told you. Shrimp mousse! Molded into a lovely lobster."

Now Shelly's beeper was going off. She grabbed for it on the bedside table, missed and knocked it to the floor along with my keys to the office and the hospital.

"I've got to call in!" she exclaimed bolting out of bed naked. She batted her eyes.

"Well, there's not quite thirty," Mrs. Van Schench continued. "Let's see, two couples declined. That's twenty-six. Then there's the Senator and the maid--I don't know if she ate any mousse--oh, you didn't? Lucy doesn't eat mousse--oh, I'm sorry Lucy--Lucy doesn't like being called a *maid*--and the black Labrador retriever, Joe, he got into it. Well, he really didn't *get* into it. We gave him the damaged claw. We can't find Joe. And poor Miss Penny has lain down and *died* on the kitchen tiles. Oh, it's simply horrible." There was a dramatic pause before she continued with muted hysteria. "Miss Penny climbed on a chair and was on the counter eating the mousse when Lucy and I found her. We put her out and spooned out the part she'd ruined for Joe."

"The mousse?"

"Just the part Miss Penny ate from."

"You went ahead and served the mousse?"

"I had to, don't you see. I didn't have anything else. They loved it; it was such a success, garnished with parsley and paprika. I used black olives for the little eyes. Even without the claw they oohed and ahhed. I can't possibly tell them I served them mousse after the dog had been in it. Oh, it's a scandal," she sobbed.

"I can't hear you," I said.

Mrs. Van Schench told Lucy to close the door to the dining room and turn up the dinner music. "You'll just have to tell them something when you arrive to pump them out. Can't you just pretend something contaminated the water?"

"How long has it been since your guests ate the mousse?" I could hear the theme from "Chariots of Fire" in the background.

"Let's see. We served the beef course precisely at nine. We were clearing the table for dessert when we found Miss Penny, who came in through the pet door and dropped dead, after throwing up blood, of course. Boss Richardson, Mrs. Dearborn, and my other guests have been poisoned now for a little over an hour."

"How about *you*?" I asked. "How do you feel?" Mrs. Van Schench was a flake, but I thought she'd shown real courage not to panic.

"I feel dreadful," she said, "but of course I didn't eat any mousse. How could I, after seeing Miss Penny eating off the plate? Dogs carry germs in their saliva, don't they? Or is that cats?"

"O.K. listen. I can't pump out thirty people. I don't even have a stomach pump in the ambulance."

"Twenty-five," she reminded me. "Two couples regretted and I didn't eat any shrimp mousse. Doctor, what are you doing in the ambulance?"

"Never mind that. Listen, you're going to have to purge their stomachs right away. I'll get there as soon as I can. Do you have any Ipecac?"

"What's that?"

"Never mind, do you have any hydrogen peroxide?" I'd learned from Dr. Hartwell, the vet, that doses over 10% could cause burning, but that over-the-counter hydrogen peroxide was three percent. It wasn't used as an emetic, except for dogs.

There was no LD .50 on the relative toxicity of hydrogen peroxide, and Hartwell had assured me that a 30cc dose would cause no side effects other than a foaming up of the stomach contents and violent purgation. The fact that Miss Penny had regurgitated blood worried me that the poodle had gotten into some rat poison containing Warfarin or Coumadin, although taken orally, rat poison should have taken longer to kill even a small dog. The dog could have gotten poisoned independent of the shrimp mousse, but I was afraid to take a chance. Bad seafood was dangerous. No matter what, the worst that could happen was I could ruin the Van Schench supper party and my dubious reputation. I decided that the most prudent thing to do was to empty everybody's stomach.

"Yes, I think I have hydrogen peroxide in the medicine cabinet."

"Is Ida Worthy there?" Ida was the only person I could think of who might be able to coerce twenty-five people and Senator Boss Richardson into drinking hydrogen peroxide.

"Of course, the commissioner and Mrs. Worthy are both here. Everybody who is anybody at *all* is here."

Shelly was standing in a frozen lurch in the middle of the floor blinking her eyes.

"Good! Is Melody Clayton, the pharmacist, there?"

"No."

"Hartwell, the vet?"

"No."

"A nurse, maybe?"

"We didn't invite the, ah, medical community. But I plan to have another party very soon and invite you all. I've been wanting do something nice for that handsome Dr. Maloy and all of your associates." I couldn't picture Margaret Holt agreeing to go to a supper party at the Van Schench mansion.

"Never mind that," I said. "Put Ida Worthy on."

"I've got to call in," Shelly said. She'd put on my lab coat without buttoning it up, and she was frozen in mid-step.

I cupped the receiver. "I think this is the emergency right here. Claudia Van Schench has poisoned *everybody-who-is-anybody* plus her poodle and black lab." Shelly's buzzer went off again, and Ida Worthy's husky voice answered loudly. I heard Claudia urging her to whisper.

"Whisper hell," boomed Ida. "Whisper and call hogs! I forgot how to whisper fifty years ago! Well, Otis, what can I do for you besides whisper you up some sweet-talk on Claudia's goddamn sterling silver telephone."

"Listen carefully, Miss Ida. Claudia says there was something wrong with the shrimp mousse you had for dinner."

"Me?"

"Y'all," I corrected.

"Not me," said Ida. "You won't catch me eating no damn fish Jello. I never started."

"Good," I said. "Ida, you've got to get everybody outside and make them drink some hydrogen peroxide."

"How much?" At least one person in Grady trusted my judgment. There was no more suspicion in Ida's voice than if I'd asked her to pass the grits.

"About 30 cc's. One ounce. Use a whiskey jigger. Measure out an ounce and give everybody a shot. Can you persuade Boss Richardson to help you round everybody up and get them outside?"

"Malcolm? Has a baboon got a ass?"

"Like a Canadian sunset," I chuckled. "And Ida, remember when I asked you how to grow kudzu?"

"I got you, Doc. Toss it down and step back."

"Fine. Oh, if you see the Van Schench's black lab, give him a shot too. I'm on my way. Be there in twenty minutes."

Shelly called the ER. Buster told her that Mrs. Van Schench called in an emergency, but wouldn't state the nature of the emergency.

We dressed and jumped into the ambulance, howling through the mild December night. "Watch out!" I screamed as we topped a hill, "somebody's stopped in the road. A pickup was sideways across the centerline. Shelly slammed on the brakes and the big ambulance squatted as it slowed, swerving around the truck. "Isn't that Frog Hullet?" I asked. We were within a quarter mile of the Van Schenchs' address. Frog was standing in the headlights holding a shotgun broken at the breach and staring into the ditch.

"He's been firelighting," Shelly said. "He's blinded a raccoon or deer with his headlights and killed it, the son-of-a-bitch. I'm calling the game warden." The ambulance swerved as she scribbled Frog's tag number and radioed the Law Enforcement Office of the Department of Natural Resources. "If it's a deer, they'll confiscate his gun and his truck. It'll serve the dirty-leg bastard right. You take a pick-up truck and a gun away from a redneck, all you've got left is white trash."

The siren wound down as we traveled the long driveway to the Van Schenchs' white-columned antebellum mansion. Ida Worthy was standing at the side of the house waving to us with a large plastic syringe with a rubber bulb on the end.

"What's that?" I asked Shelly as we jogged across the lawn.

"Turkey baster."

"That's what it looks like. Or an enema."

"It's a turkey baster."

We rounded the corner of the house into the back yard where twenty-five people, including Boss Richardson and Mildred Hesse, bent at the waist heaving, puffing vapor, and regurgitating shrimp mousse, beef stroganoff, and foam into the boxwood topiaries and flower beds. Claudia Van Schench strolled among them, passing out tissues from a sterling silver dispenser. Lucy followed her with a roll of toilet paper.

"Looks like you've got everything under control here, Ida," I acknowledged, "but what's the turkey baster for?"

"Some of these folks, including the lab, didn't want to drink no peroxide," she said. "But we got some into everbody all the same. The lab, he run off after he got his dose."

"I'm ruined," lamented Claudia Van Schench. "Ruined." Boss Richardson, a born leader, was barking orders even as bubbles escaped from his nose and mouth.

Holly Meyers, an uninvited neighbor from the next block, rounded the house.

"Oh Claudia, I'm so sorry. I've been trying to call you. At first the line was busy. Then nobody answered. I've been *frantic*."

"Oh, what do *you* want, Holly?" she sighed. "Can't you see I'm simply devastated?"

Holly was astounded by the behavior of Mrs. Van Schench's guests. Her jaw dropped, and she pressed her palm beneath her neck. "I ran over Miss Penny with the car! She ran away, but she's hurt. I tried to catch her to take her to Dr. Hartwell, but she disappeared." Her eyes were fixed on Mildred Hesse, who bent over a boxwood and barked like a seal. "I've looked everywhere," Holly continued. "She didn't come home, did she? I'm so, so, sorry. She just ran right out so fast that her little paws were all a-blur, and there was absolutely *nothing* I could do to avoid her. Oh, I could feel the bumpy-bump of the tire as it rolled over poor, poor Miss Penny!"

Claudia's chin dropped to her strand of oriental pearls. "You *what*?"

"Your poodle! I've accidentally run over your dog. I'm so *sorry*."

"Me too," said Frog Hullet, stepping up like a water bird and removing his baseball cap. "If your name's Van Something-or-other and you live at this here address, I just shot your black lab--Joe Van Something-or-other, it said on the collar."

"My dog?" Claudia mumbled, in shock. She had a thousand-yard stare. "Why would anybody shoot my dog?"

"Well, he come running down the middle of the road foaming out the mouth. I hate I had to be the one to kill him."

184

"Who," she said absently, "are you?"

"Mister Maynard Hullet," Frog said, grinning and stepping forward, holding out his hand, "but you can call me Frog." Mrs. Van Schench did not shake hands with Frog. She stood dumbfounded. "I went on and cut off his head. Animal control people will want his head. I brung you his collar. The rest of him's in the ditch down the road. I'll help your husband dig a hole, you want me to. I don't 'spect he's dressed to bury no dog."

"Let's get out of here," I told Shelly, "before anybody else recognizes us." Karl Wright, wiping his face with a silk handkerchief, danced backwards to avoid soiling his shoes. The game warden's green truck was pulling in behind Frog's pickup as we left, its blue flasher pulsing into the darkness.

"Merry Christmas," I told Shelly as she started the ambulance. "Now you know how the other half lives. Everybody-who-is-anybody blows lunch just like us common folks."

"Morton Willetts was there, barfing into the verbena and foaming like a crab," she said. "I smell a malpractice suit."

"Miss Ida made him drink the peroxide. He'll have to come through her to get to me."

"If Miss Ida's running interference, I'd say you've got pretty good field position."

"Will you marry me if I get Miss Ida to be the maid of honor or the flower girl?"

"I might," said Shelly. "I just might."

Chapter Forty

I'm picking you up," Rooster Bootman growled into the telephone. "Be out front."

"What's wrong?" I said.

"Two cars in a head-on out 85."

"Why don't you send the ambulance?"

"Did. The ambulance run off the James Pond bridge."

My knees weakened, my stomach tightened. I found myself holding on to Early May's desk for support. "Call the hospital," I croaked. "See who's out."

My emergency pack was hanging on the hat rack. One of Early May's self-imposed duties was to make sure the medical supplies in the pack were replenished and serviceable. She handed it to me as she called the dispatcher and verified what I already knew. Shelly wasn't going to be left behind when there was a head-on. There was the psychological baggage of saving her parents. She was the best too, the most highly qualified, in spite of or because of all that baggage.

"Shelly and Buster!" Early May cried. I snatched up my pack and rushed past Thomas Freelander, who was laying bricks as his grandson played in the sand. Rooster's patrol car was bucking down the street, lights flashing and siren moaning and squalling. On the way to the James Pond Bridge I tried to compose myself, wringing my hands, grilling Rooster with staccato questions he couldn't answer.

"How many injured in the head-on?"

"Didn't say."

"What caused the ambulance to wreck?"

"Don't know."

"Did whoever called say anything about a girl--about Shelly?"

"Not to me." Bootman contacted Melvin Dryden on the radio, telling him to bring the wrecker and to ask Bill Worthy to come out or send somebody in a pickup with the camper shell. "And don't you bust your ass getting out here," Bootman added. Buster Hogue and Melvin Dryden were both notoriously fast drivers. They grew up during a time when official vehicles with flashing lights were supposed to speed. The drama of squalling tires and screeching sirens had drawn them to their respective professions.

The highway made a long curve before the bridge crossed, side-by-side with the railroad trestle, the tannin-tinted water of James Pond. The guardrail was open where the ambulance had torn through, and a yellow mongrel dog lay broken and dead on the double yellow line. There was an eerie absence of human life.

I jumped out of the car, staring down into the dark water. Immediately I saw the back of the ambulance, four feet beneath the surface, where it had nose-dived to the bottom. The cavernous dark of an open back door made me hope that the vehicle was empty, but there was no one either on the banks or in the water. The haunting red letters on the side of the vehicle wavered beneath the rippled surface like smeared lipstick. The thought of losing Shelly was abhorrent, unsustainable. I began gasping. "Maybe somebody's already taken them in. Maybe Commissioner Worthy got here with the camper before we did."

"Naw," said the sheriff, "They're over yonder."

Suddenly I heard distant human voices. I ran to the other side of the bridge and saw the group of motley survivors on the brown sand bank between the bridge and the trestle.

A woman lay on the ground, covered to the neck with a poncho. A man with a bloody or muddy face and a splinted arm was squatted on the concrete sandbags that banked the bridge and trestle, holding an infant swaddled in an Army fatigue jacket. Another man with dry trousers and shirtless stood by a beached jonboat talking with a teenage boy in a neck brace, but my eyes fell first upon what they searched for the hardest: a drenched figure of a girl in a muddy white and magenta uniform, walking in circles and beating her clenched fists against her thighs, stamping her foot--the familiar gestures of rage and frustration of my beloved Shelly.

But my relief was tempered by the realization that Buster Hogue wasn't with her.

Down the highway past the bridge there was a dirt path that fishermen used to launch their boats. Back in the patrol car, Bootman and I followed it to the survivors. I jumped out before he could stop, running to Shelly, hugging her, holding her soaked body against mine and pressing my cheek against her cold, wet hair. "Buster's trapped in there!" she screamed. "He's stuck between the cab and the back. Oh Otis! He tried to crawl through to help, and he drowned! He drowned! Oh Otis, Buster drowned!" Her face was pale, her eyes bloodshot from tears and muddy water.

She was frustrated and crushed and bawling, but she was not hysterical. Her patients were taken care of. The teenaged boy in the neck brace had one arm splinted ingeniously with a life jacket and a length of anchor rope borrowed from the fisherman. "I broke my neck when I had a blow-out and run into them folks," he explained. "I broke my arm in the ambulance wreck,"

Shelly told me the infant wasn't hurt, that everybody was ready to transport, but I should see about the woman, give her morphine. I examined the woman. Inflated MAST trousers supported a fractured hip.

"That girl over yonder, she saved my wife and baby," the husband began, smiling weakly. "Me, I sidestroked on out with a broke arm, but that girl there, she's the one got my woman and my baby girl out."

Much later, Shelly was able to tell me what happened. After the ambulance had crashed into the pond, it floated nose down for awhile before it filled with water and dove to the bottom. Shelly unstraped the woman and her husband from their stretchers and ordered the teenager, in spite of his broken arm, to climb onto the husband's shoulders and open a back door.

Buster had tried to squirm through the small opening between the cab and the back, a tight fit even for Shelly. "Go out through the front!" she'd screamed, "and swim around!" But already the water had risen to Buster's neck. One arm reached out to Shelly. The other was pinned at the shoulder. "Grab my legs!" she cried, squatting over Buster's head, knowing that his one arm was stronger than she could be. She held the infant with one arm and pulled Buster's arm with the other until the dark water rose above his ears. "Buster," she screamed "let the air out of your lungs, collapse your chest and wiggle through." She scissored his distorted face between her knees, tugging him with her thighs as the water rose. She felt his struggling head between her legs as the water covered her lap, his head bubbling, his hand clawing at her as she squeezed his face beneath her thighs, tugging with all her strength, crying, praying, cursing as the water rose. She had to let Buster go to keep the unconscious woman's head above the rising water as the inflated MAST splint floated her hips, threatening to invert her. She felt Buster's hand grasp her ankle and hold her back until the last moment when she herself was gasping. Then Buster released her, and her heart felt him drown.

Shelly had supported the mother's head on her shoulder and held the child as the MAST trousers floated them up the vertical walls of the ambulance, through the narrow door, out into the sunlight.

When the fisherman got to them, she handed him the infant and held to the gunnels of the jonboat and to the floating woman while he idled to shore, keeping the mother's broken bones stabilized in the water.

I sent Shelly to the hospital with Bill Worthy and the injured. Rooster and I waited for Melvin and the wrecker. I'd forgotten my windbreaker but discovered I didn't need it. It was January, but we'd had nearly a week of warm sunny days. Luckily, the water was chilly but not cold enough to cause hypothermia to the victims. We could thank God for a mild Georgia winter--at least a few days of it.

"Do you think we ought to call the volunteer fire department?" I asked Bootman. Underwater rescue was their responsibility.

"Naw, Melvin's a fireman. If he's got enough cable we'll get the ambulance in. I reckon Buster's in it. If he ain't, we'll get somebody to come out and drag. Buster's the only one in Grady can use the SCUBA"

"That's some little woman in them wine colored britches," the fisherman said. Still shirtless, his thin torso was white as mozzarella cheese until it met the sharp lines on his arms and his neck, a farmer's tan. He wore a blue baseball cap and had a triangular space between his front incisors.

"You got that right!" said Rooster Bootman.

"Well, I got to go on to the house," said the fisherman.

"Hold off," said Rooster. "After I get a statement, I want you to do me a favor. When the wrecker gets here, see if you can't run out there and hook us up to the bumper."

"That bumper's under the water," the fisherman said.

"Well, I'll send a fireman out there with you to hook up," Rooster said.

When Melvin arrived, there was a brief dispute over who was going to get in the water to hook up the cable. Melvin said he wasn't in the underwater rescue section of the volunteer fire department--that was Buster's job. Besides, he had to operate the winch and drive the wrecker.

The fisherman and Rooster couldn't swim, or said they couldn't, so the task fell upon me. There wasn't enough cable to pull the ambulance from the bank, so Melvin lowered the hook off the bridge for me and the fisherman to motor out and attach to the sunken vehicle. I stripped to my baby blue UNC Tarheels bikini underwear Shelly had ordered as a novelty gift and hopped into the boat. As luck would have it, they were the only clean underwear in my drawer. I'd never worn them before.

"Is that the kind of shorts Yankees wear?" Rooster wanted to know.

I grinned sheepishly. "A gift," I said.

"Whooee!" said Melvin, grateful for some comic relief. He couldn't say anything without his voice breaking. He and Buster had been buddies since grammar school.

The January air was chilly but not cold as we motored out to the ambulance. The water temperature, however, had a definite sting. I was able to stand on the one closed door in water up to my waist, but I had to duck under to reach the bumper. I had to swim under more than once, holding my breath and trying to get the hook to bite into something. Each time I dove and struggled to make the cable fast, my buttocks bobbed to the surface, and by the time I had made the hook fast a small heterogenous crowd of men, women, and children had gathered, some of whom cheered--either for my success with the attachment or in facetious celebration of my derriere. I couldn't see well enough underwater to find Buster.

Melvin drove slowly along the bridge. The cable vibrated as he dragged the heavy ambulance toward the shore. When it got to the water's edge, he let off on the cable and I unhooked it. He drove the wrecker down a dirt path to the water's edge, and I reattached the cable to the rear bumper, quickly jumped into my trousers, and threw on my shirt before the crowd, hungry for drama, joined me on the sandy beach.

The winch pulled the ambulance up the steep bank. The cable moaned.

"See can you open a front door and let the water out faster," Melvin called. "I'm bogging down."

Rooster opened the driver's door and the water gushed out. From where I stood looking in the back door, a huge bubble broke to the surface and the water drained quickly, but it didn't wash Buster out, and I was glad. He was still caught chest deep in the crawlspace. When the flushing water drained past him, it was as though he'd burst wide-eyed to the surface then bowed his head modestly in death as the slow winch dragged the ambulance onto the muddy strand.

Chapter Forty-One

The Feds were making us work hard for these Community Health Center dollars. One of the stipulations of the grant was for us to combine our efforts with a group of citizens who were setting up a clinic in south Flint, about 25 miles from Grady. This was going to involve some difficult politics, and since the most powerfully connected physician in the south Flint community was Dr. Gordon Powell, a black surgeon, I sent Maloy as an emissary.

Jesseanne Lockwood had mailed us a print-out of the physicians that would be at the National Health Service Corps convention at the downtown Marriott in Atlanta. Since our grant would be accepted, we were eligible to recruit. We screened and telephoned the candidates we wanted. Then we team-tagged them at the convention, which was like the TV program "Supermarket Sweep." We birddogged two internists, two pediatricians, and two physician's assistants (PA's) to staff the Grady and South Flint clinics, fed them $50 meals at Anthony's, and sold them on the idea of coming to South Georgia.

Numerous initiatives supported our goals. A new medical school was being started at Mercer University to train rural physicians. Organizations such as the National Rural Health Association and the National Association of Community Health Centers were being formed to address the plight of the rural poor. Help was coming, but we knew this scheme wasn't worth gully dirt unless we could get the new recruits hospital privileges at Putnam Memorial. I was depending on Gordon Powell's political clout at the hospital and in the community at large.

Jim came back enthusiastic from his visit with Dr. Powell. "Gordon says he'll help us."

"Gordon?" I said. "Are you already on a first name basis with Dr. Powell?"

"Sure, he's quite a guy."

I already knew without meeting Gordon Powell that he was quite a guy. He, Dr. Jeff Roberts the thoracic surgeon, and Roberts' associate Dr. Wayne Friedmon had authored a paper entitled "Peripheral Vascular Disease in Blacks." Basically the work established that amputation was a more likely coincidence in blacks than in whites during treatment of atherosclerosis because blacks have smaller vessels. The doctors found positive results through refined microvascular surgical techniques.

Gordon Powell had commanded MASH units in Korea and Viet Nam; he returned to Flint, his hometown, to improve the health care availability for blacks and indigent whites. There were few black doctors in Flint, and he worked long hours treating charity patients. He liked the idea of a federally subsidized clinic in south Flint. He also agreed to operate on one of my patients, a forty-year-old black female with a breast tumor and no insurance. Through Maloy, he invited me to scrub in and observe and to discuss politics regarding our health center. The next day his office confirmed our appointment in the Putnam OR the following Thursday.

I drove over to Putnam in Maloy's and my communal white Falcon that the Maloys had come to call *Rocinante*, in honor of our zealous, sometimes quixotic quest to save Grady from trauma and disease.

I didn't have any trouble recognizing Dr. Powell, the only black doctor in the doctors' lounge. He greeted me cheerfully, introducing me to an orthopedic surgeon who was reading the Wall Street Journal. Powell was a squat, bald man in his sixties with a wide mustached mouth and ears tilted slightly from his temples to accommodate eyeglasses. He had a distinguished yet friendly air, and he conveyed the impression that he was highly charged and motivated. He was already dressed in his green scrub suit except for hat and mask.

He led me to the doctors' locker room, where I changed and shared his locker. Then we visited the patient to reassure her and answer any questions she might have before the anesthesiologist put her under. Mattie Reynolds was a large woman with a sad smile. "I'm in your hands, Doctor," she said looking directly at me.

"Not me, Mattie," I stammered. "Dr. Powell is the surgeon. I'm just, uh, observing."

"Yes suh, you watch over him, make sure he don't do nothin wrong."

I tried to protest. I wanted Mattie to know how highly esteemed were the skills of her surgeon. I tried to tell her that I was going to be standing behind Dr. Powell, staying out of the way, but Dr. Powell quieted me by touching my arm.

As we scrubbed, Dr. Powell was cordial. He wanted to know what a guy who had graduated second in his class at Stanford was doing in a place like Grady. "I was shanghaied when my car broke down on 85," I told him.

"What's Jim Maloy doing down here in the deep South?"

"I shanghaied *him*."

"How? You put sugar in his gas tank?"

"He's married to my sister. She threatened to cut him off. Also, we're friends, med school roommates."

"He's a gregarious young fellow, isn't he?" Dr. Powell smiled. With his wet hands raised, he pushed open the double doors of the OR with his back. I followed.

"You got that right!" I laughed.

"There's a great deal of work to be done here," he said with prophetic gravity. He pushed his wet hands into the latex gloves the scrub nurse held open for him.

You sure said a mouthful there, doctor, I thought.

The patient was prepared. Dr. Powell introduced me to the anesthetist and a scrub nurse with sexy eyes. Then he made a neat half-moon incision with his scalpel around the edge of the nipple's areolae, exposing the honey-colored fatty tissue of the patient's right breast. He followed with his bovie, cutting and cauterizing, filling the air with the smell of singed flesh, as he probed for the tumor. "So while you were waiting for your car to be repaired, you occupied your time by going into private practice and opening a couple of clinics. That makes sense."

"Well, at first I was going to stay just long enough to help Dr. Hogue get Trafford on its feet. When Dr. Hogue dropped dead, I couldn't just abandon his patients and mine too. After that, one thing led to another."

"The way I see it, you can help me by reducing my work load of indigent patients. I'll pay you back by operating for free on your patients who can't afford to pay."

"Is it a deal?" I asked hopefully.

"Well, you can count on my cooperation," he said, cutting deeper with short strokes of the bovie, which hissed and spit and smoked. He hooked the incision apart with his thumbs. "My associates and I feel an obligation to see all patients regardless of insurance status, but you have some reason to be concerned about how well your health centers will be received in the community. The winds of change are blowing down here. There is a group of us who believe in upholding the Putnam Memorial ethic of seeing all who need to be seen, but we're threatened on all sides. HMO's are being started in Atlanta. They're targeting large statewide agencies like the school system and Federal Employees. Here in Flint we have Karl Wright who is building a private, for-profit system. Hell, Karl even plans to sell preferred stock. I'm afraid if we aren't careful, our health care system will become two-tiered--one for the rich and one for the poor. In the deep South we are all too familiar with separate and unequal. If Putnam converts to private for-profit, you'll have to ship your indigent patients to Augusta, about four hours from here."

Tiny orts of spongy tan fat lay on the green cloth cover under the patient's chin. Powell, his elbows raised, removed a small, sausage-shaped tumor with forceps and dropped it into a stainless steel kidney-shaped pan. "Take this to the pathologist," he told the scrub nurse with the bright eyes.

"Yes," he told me. "I guess it's a deal. Your heart seems to be in the right place, even if your brains aren't."

"Uh, and there's one other thing."

"Tell me." Dr. Powell said. He inserted his index finger knuckle-deep into the incision feeling around for another mass.

"I need political clout to set up the south Flint clinic,"
I said.

"Um, hum, you surely do, and some help to run it."

I told him we had recruited two more internists, two peds, and two PA's from
the National Health Service Corps. Our first choice was to recruit family
physicians, but they were in ridiculously short supply. "And I'll need some help
making reciprocal arrangements with other Flint doctors," I added.

"Yes, you will. You'll be on salary, and to most of my reactionary colleagues,
being on salary is equivalent to being a communist."

"I'll be accepted as a volunteer in the National Health Service Corps,
commissioned as light Colonel at $32,000," I told him. "I'll also need somebody
like you to make sure Putnam Memorial will accept Medicaid, Medicare, and
indigent patients from the clinics. We're not going to dump on the local doctors.
We'll admit and manage our own patients. We'll ask for help only when we
absolutely have to, and we'll be available for consultation with other doctors
whether their patients have any money or not."

"That's more than *one* thing."

"Well, my heart's in the right place."

"So it seems." Dr. Powell was closing up, sewing the patient's purplish nipple
back on, pushing the tiny fang-shaped sutures through the lips of the incision,
which he closed with dark thread.

"Do you happen to know a 'good ole boy' down your way named Hack
Singletree?" Powell tilted his head to examine his needlework.

"Sure! Hack's a friend of mine. Do you know him?"

"Sure, I hunt quail on Toa Plantation two or three times a year with him. Give
him my regards if you see him and mind this advice: No matter how drunk Mr.
Singletree may seem, do not shoot against him for money or other items of
consideration."

"You sound experienced."

"Have you ever heard of a field trials champion named Gordy Pow?"

"Sure, that's Hack's liverspot English."

"Gordy Pow was my inadvertent contribution to Singletree Kennels," Dr.
Powell said as we pushed through the swinging doors of the OR and returned to
the lounge.

"Small world," I exclaimed, pulling down my mask.

"The world's not so small, but southwest Georgia is."

————————

The next week Dr. Powell and Paul Dudley showed up with Dr. Thomas
Ling, medical director of the National Association of Community Health

Centers. Since their visit coincided with a visit from one of our recruited pediatricians and the two P.A.'s, Hack commandeered a school bus to show them around. We toured Flint's southside, where one of our clinics would be located, and spent a few morning hours at Putnam Memorial. Then we dropped off Powell and Dudley and rattled around locations of medical and cultural interest in Grady, which after Trafford, the clinic, and the health department, took about 15 min. Dr. Ling above all else wanted to see an alligator. Born in Hawaii, Ling was an affable Asian American with bright bookish eyes. He was excited by nearly everything we showed him, snapping pictures with the Instamatic and Minolta cameras that hung around his neck. "Isn't that interesting?" said Ling when we showed him a soul food cafe in south Flint. He must have taken three dozen pictures of cypress knees.

"There ain't a lot of alligators out in January," said Hack, "but there's a pretty good one likes to sun off the west bank of James Pond. We might can get a look at him." I knew the surface of James Pond wasn't frigid. I'd been swimming in it once already this month hooking a wrecker cable to our ambulance. Hack quipped alligators were more thin-skinned and climate-sensitive than carpetbaggers, adding that there was a shallow bayou that warmed up suitably for alligators by this time of day. We banged down the dirt road that led along the shore of the pond. Dr. Ling perched on the edge of his naugahyde seat taking in the scenery with quick birdlike glances while hanging on for dear life to the back of the driver's seat as the bus bounced over potholes and washes. The pediatrician and the P.A.'s, having little interest in alligators but being well aware of Ling's importance to their professional future, tolerated the ride with white-knuckle grips on the backs of the bench seats in front of them. Still they slid and bounced, clenching their teeth to keep from clacking down on their tongues.

"Move on up front and you won't ride so rough!" Hack yelled over his shoulder. His face was broken up in the large rear view mirror like ripples on the pond. It didn't occur to him to slow the bus down. Of course, the medical personnel in the back of the bus couldn't move anywhere until he did. They'd bank around like pinballs if they attempted the slightest maneuver. The rear axle dropped into a gully wash bucking a P.A. nearly to the vaulted metal ceiling. Ling was enjoying every bump. He even tried to take photographs out the windows, hanging on like a spider monkey with one hand.

Finally we pulled over on a grassy bank and Hack pointed out what he said was an eight-foot alligator among the lilypads. The reptile was completely submerged except for the knob of its nose and the knot of one eye in profile. It could have been a log for all we knew. It could have been anything until almost imperceptibly it moved, swaying its slow tail, making a thin silver ripple in the onyx water. Ling fired a flurry of pictures, none of which could possibly have been distinguishable as an alligator.

Hack pulled me aside. "Why's he so fascinated by alligators?"

"I don't know. He's fascinated by a lot of things."

"Not like a damn alligator, which is about all he's talked about since he got off the plane. It must be they put him to mind of dragons. Dragons play big with them people."

"What people?"

"A Chinaman."

"He's an American," I reminded Hack, who grinned.

"Well, his America is a right smart piece away from mine, but if he's so important to your cause and all, I reckon we need to get him a respectable picture of that alligator to take back to Hawaii."

"He lives in Washington."

"I'd heap rather live in Hawaii." He waved his arms, making signs with his fingers and rotating his hips, like a hula dancer. Then with his forearm still raised and his hand angled horizontal like a swan's head, he marched over to Dr. Ling, who was putting a new role of film in the Minolta. "A alligator lays like this in the water," he told Ling, "and he sinks backwards. He lets out his air, and his tail pulls him down."

"Isn't that interesting?" said Dr. Ling.

"If a gator sunk forward," he continued, "you could get you a noose and catch ever one in Georgia."

Ling nodded enthusiastically. "Is there any way I can get a photograph of an alligator," he asked, "without a telephoto lens."

"Well, you can wait till that one crawls up on the bank. Or you can get somebody to haul his ass up for you."

Dr. Ling smiled widely. "You?"

"I'm about the best there is." Hack sat on the steps of the bus, removing his brogans and socks and rolling up his trousers. "You aren't thinking about wading out there after that alligator," I said.

"Why Doc, catching a gator is about the easiest thing in the world."

"He'll never hold still."

"Naw, he'll go to the bottom, where he'll think I can't see him."

"He'll bite you."

"Naw, I'll get him around the neck and hold his mouth shut. A gator can bust a bowling ball when he chomps down, but you can hold his mouth shut with two fingers." He held up a thumb and index finger as though conducting a last minute inspection of his gator grabbing equipment. Then he took his flask, keys, and billfold from his pockets, nesting them into his Stetson, which he handed to me. Now he had the everyone's attention. Dr. Ling scurried around measuring light, making sure he had plenty of film in both cameras.

Hack tiptoed into the water and began moving slowly toward the alligator, so slowly that his movement was nearly imperceptible. By the time he was crotch deep in the pond, he seemed an inanimate snag among the lily pads. His stalk was best described as reptilian. "To catch an alligator," I explained, "you have to think like one. Which takes awhile since alligators have a brain the size of a peanut." I was a little piqued at Hack for setting out on this improbable venture when we had to get to the Flint airport for the 5:47 shuttle to Atlanta. I was angry with myself for allowing Hack to start such a project, as if I had any control over him whatsoever when a bright idea dawned. I guessed I shouldn't be too mad since he was trying to impress Ling for me. Of course, Hack didn't have any more regard for catching the 5:47 than the alligator did.

My medical entourage began glancing at wristwatches, except for Dr. Ling, who leaned over, hands on knees, totally absorbed in a scene that was all but static. From time to time he checked his light meter, readjusting to the lengthening shadows and declining sun.

When Hack had progressed about three-quarters of the way to the alligator, a white cattle egret with yellow beak and legs lit with a squawk between the horny charcoal knobs of the alligator's eyes. It remained long enough for Ling to click off a few frames with the Instamatic before realizing the deadly nature of its perch. It suddenly launched into the air like a pinwheel, shedding downfeathers and squawking hysterically as though outraged by a reality that *seems* but is not. And what the hell was that *human* doing out here, leaning over in waist deep water so that only the dark head and wide back inched through the waxy lily pads.

"What's he going to do when he gets out there," one of the P.A.'s yawned. Like many of the first physicians assistants, this one had been a medic in Viet Nam and wasn't easily impressed. The other, also a former medic, had crawled back into the school bus to take a nap. The pediatrician unscrewed the cap on Hack's flask. He smelled the neck and made a horrible face. "Want to sample some stump?" I inquired. He didn't.

"When he gets close enough," I improvised to the P.A., "he'll try to lock one arm around the gator's neck. That way he'll be out of reach of the jaws and safe from the tail." I was doing pretty good. Ling, although he didn't take his eyes off the alligator and Hack, cocked an ear toward every syllable. "At first he'll just hang on and let the alligator thrash around and tire out. They're very powerful creatures, but they don't have much stamina." There was a long, quizzical silence. "He'll tilt the nose up," I added, "so the gator will swim to the surface. Holding their head back makes them sleepy too."

Even Dr. Ling's expression was dubious. "Isn't that interesting?" he said. "Hack can hold his breath underwater a long time," I assured them.

Hack was less than ten feet from the alligator when it submerged. Hack disappeared immediately after, and we held our breath and watched the gentle ripples on the surface until suddenly it exploded as the alligator breached the water, rising on its powerful tail, slinging foam like a marlin, black as a tractor tire except for its creamy throat and underside. Hack was still aboard, his legs running in mid air, before disappearing again into the dark water. The second time they surfaced, they were closer to shore, as though Hack were indeed bulldogging the reptile towards us, although it was obvious by his wide eyes that he wasn't in absolute control. His head alone sped along the surface, his nose prowing a V through the water, making a twin wake behind his swept back hair. Ling and the others stood on the bank, their mouths agape. His cameras swung uselessly from his neck. Suddenly there was a terrific eruption and a wall of water as the gator lashed its tail, slinging Hack into the air. The gator followed Hack, who ran through the shallow water like a threshing machine, falling into the mud at Ling's feet, then scrambling on all fours toward the bus as the alligator crawled halfway out of the water. It arched its back, opening its white mouth and hissing like an air compressor. Ling, backpedaling, snapped a picture with the Instamatic.

Hack squirmed to a sitting position holding his arm. "You all right?" I asked.

"He must've wrenched my arm," he said. He propped his chin in his hand and worked his jaw. "He must've wrenched my jaw too."

"I'm impressed," I said. Actually, I was relieved that I hadn't lost another friend to James Pond in the same month.

"Nothing to it. Like I said, catching an alligator is about the easiest thing in the world."

"Well, what's the hardest thing."

"The hardest thing," he grinned, "is turning one of the sumbitches a-loose."

"Wasn't that interesting?" beamed Dr. Ling. "I wish I could have gotten a closeup with the Minolta."

"Do it again, Hack," I said.

Chapter Forty-Two

W e got tax revenues of $3,600,000," began Chairman Bill Worthy around his unlit cheroot, which jutted like a dark handle for his bald, round head. I'd ordered him to quit smoking but couldn't wean him from his cigar. The best he'd do was leave his matches at home. As chairman of the County Commission, he'd called an emergency meeting of commissioners and the hospital authority. I was there in my official capacity as chief of staff of the hospital, as the only physician on the authority, and as the medical advisor to the EMT service. Maloy was at work, where he belonged. "Twenty-five percent of that goes for health," Worthy continued, "so we got $900,000 to split up between Trafford, the Health Department, and the ambulance. That's four-hundred thou for Trafford--three for health and two for the meat wagon, which presently is down at Melvin's with mud in the cylinders. Much as I hate it, something's got to go. Anderson here tells me he's going to need $600,000 to $700,000 for Trafford. Shelly needs two thousand, after we get a new ambulance, which will cost $75,000. Mrs. Rhodes at the Health Department needs her $200,000. The auditors tell us we got more medicine than the county can afford. Something's got to go down the tube."

I'd known this was coming. Before Maloy arrived, the hospital was losing $40,000 a month. Now, even with its revenues increased, it was still losing $20,000. Before Hogue's death Trafford was breaking even, but as Anderson and nearly everybody else had told me, "Doc Hogue kept Trafford slap full of babies and appendectomies." Maloy and I, of course, delivered zero babies. Mrs. Rhodes at the Health Department wanted to handle prenatal care for poverty level mothers. Doctors Middlebrooks and Clasper, Flint obstetricians, had agreed to deliver our babies at Putnam until we could recruit a family physician.

The Health Department was also administrating most of the childhood immunizations and doing well-child care through the EPSDT program. There was no way we could cut out the Health Department. Without it we couldn't even license May's Oyster Bar, the only decent place in town to eat. The only place to deliver Elroy Singletree's dinner.

But we couldn't do without the hospital. Not with two internists. An internist was nothing without a hospital, although Maloy had disagreed. He felt we could do a great deal without Trafford, which he thought was a ruptured duck anyway. My response to that kind of thinking was that Maloy had lost a lot of brain cells to the Montezuma two-step. That, or Nancy had turned him into a social worker. The Maloys believed that the mere existence of a hospital caused medicine to focus on emergencies rather than prevention.

"Commissioner," I said. "I don't see how any of these essential medical services can be discontinued."

"Son, that ain't one of the options. You know if there was a way in the world to help you, we'd do it. Ain't nobody more dedicated to health care than this gaggle of folks setting right here in this courthouse. That's why we're handing you the ax, so chop. You're the doctor; you decide."

Beulah's legs were crossed at the knees. She was wiggling her foot, which must have subliminally aroused my prurient interests in recollection of her pedal shenanigans at the hospital authority meeting. Besides Beulah, the omnipresent Morton Willetts was there, propping his chin on his interlaced fingers and watching me over his glasses.

"Discontinue the EMS," I decided.

"Good decision," said Anderson. "Difficult, but good."

If it was such a good decision, why didn't I feel good?

"I know that was hard on you," Beulah confided after the meeting had adjourned. Her green eyes sparkled. "What will your poor, sweet Shelly do with herself? Will she go on to Vanderbilt now? Or will she stay here with you, feather your nest, work on her MRS-MD?"

"She'll find something," I said. "Shelly is very, uh, resilient."

"I'm sure she is," Beulah cooed. "But do you know what I've been thinking? I've been thinking that you and my husband could have something in common. You should come around."

There was only one thing in the world Lee Bob and I could possibly have in common, which was the very thing she was talking about. It was propped up by those long legs and framed by those ardent hips. Lee Bob's wife was radiating enough sexuality to water my eyes. But no thanks, lady, although your sidelong glance and provocative cleavage are making me sweat. *What is a man that he must swim in troubled waters, that havoc and the flinty heart must be his desire?*

I dreaded breaking the ambulance news to Shelly. I didn't know what I was going to say. It turned out I didn't have to say anything. I went home after my rounds and found her gone. A note on the refrigerator said goodby, she'd be in touch, love Shelly. I tried to find solace in the "love" but couldn't. I jumped in the Falcon and sped to her house, where I found one of Russell Robin's for sale signs in the yard and a lock box on the door. Russell was Grady's principal real estate broker, although one in every three citizens seemed to have a sales license. I wondered who had tipped her off for her to move so fast? Beulah? Shelly must have planned well in advance for this contingency. The decision to discontinue the ambulance hadn't been made until ten this morning, less than twelve hours before I came home to her note.

I rushed home to call Nancy, who hadn't talked to Shelly. Then I called Russell Robin. "Hallooo," he answered. Russell wore spiked hair and a bow tie. Over the telephone his voice was indistinguishable from Hooks, the funeral director. "Nooo, it's very strange," he said. "Shelly instructed me over the telephone. She came by the office to sign the listing agreement on her way out of town. She's selling most of her furniture with the house, but she was dragging a U-Haul."

"What? She had a car?"

"Well Doctor, she wasn't pulling it with a mule. Sure, she had a car, an old Chevrolet Impala. I believe it was dark blue or black."

Shelly hadn't told Russell where she was going, only that she wouldn't be back, not even for the closing. She said she'd be in touch. Maybe she told somebody at the bank. She'd have to withdraw her savings. But no, she wouldn't have to tell the bank anything. The U-Haul. Whoever rents U-Hauls would have to know their destination. I called Melvin Dryden. He'd rented her the trailer but had promised not to tell where she was off to. He said that he'd hooked it up to one of his rentals.

I couldn't stand the thought of Shelly going anywhere in one of Melvin's rentals, which were certified jalopies. Standard operational procedure was to take the tag off and leave it on the side of the road if it broke down at a distance greater than fifty miles. Most rentals didn't make it back, but Melvin rented them for more than they were worth, and added wrecker insurance for service within the defined area. If a rental broke down within a fifty-mile radius, Melvin would drag it back as a public service. Anything beyond that he couldn't be responsible for. The fifty miles roughly corresponded to the sum of Rooster Bootman's jurisdiction and reciprocation agreements with other sheriffs. Rooster would make Melvin pick up any car left on the side of the road in a three-county area, whether the tag was removed or not.

"When is she bringing the car back?" I asked with itchy impatience.

"She ain't. It's one of my one-ways. She can just drop it off at a junkyard where she's at. I've done made arrangements with an old boy to receive the car and take Miss Shelly where she wants to go."

"You going to be down at the garage for a while?"

"Sure, why?"

"Because I'm on the way down there to overhaul your ass unless you tell me the destination of that trailer."

"Aw Doc, it's Nashville, Tennessee, but that's all I know. To Walden's Gulf on Baker at First. And don't you tell her I told you nothing! Miss Shelly get mad, she'll hiss and piss like a panther, but I guess you already know that."

Chapter Forty-Three

I couldn't believe Shelly had left so quickly. Surely, we hadn't enjoyed optimal circumstances for a love affair. I was a Yankee, Irish Catholic with culturally chauvinistic tendencies. She was a WASP Rebel feminist, but life and love are full of minor adjustments and compromises. Shelly, who wasn't used to taking a back seat to anybody, had been progressively forced into a supportive role, but I thought she was adjusting to that. I thought we were happy, or as happy as busy people get. We'd really had only one violent quarrel, not counting the time I came in drunk and late for supper after I'd been searching the Toa for the Gatorman. The fight that took the longest to cool began as an abstract discussion concerning the distinction between Northern abrasiveness and Southerners' procrastination--their absolute refusal to get down to business before beating around an interminable bush of social platitudes and nonsense.

Arriving in Grady, I'd found the citizens' reluctance to get to the point maddening. I was even more infuriated by the fact that they labeled people who do try to get to the point, namely me, *abrupt*. When I tried to conform to the custom by avoiding the purpose of the discussion for the first few moments of conversation, they accused me of *hemming and hawing*.

"The difference is," Shelly explained in her living room one Sunday, "you hem and haw because your preliminary conversation isn't genuine." We'd just returned from Shelly's church, an ecumenical compromise. "Everybody can tell you don't really give a blistered rat's ass about the weather or how everybody's family is. People can tell you're about to rupture yourself to get to some *point*, which you think's more important than the people you're getting to the point with. It's a matter of focus."

"I don't buy that," I said. "Who really cares about the weather, anyway?" I sprawled out on her living room sofa, innocently expecting a stimulating discussion.

"The people in Grady do," she said. "*I* do. This is an agricultural community, and the weather is more important than any poignant and earthshaking *point* it could occur to you to make."

"You're getting mad. Why are you getting mad?" I asked, swinging my feet to the floor.

"Because you always miss the point, just like when you insist on calling rheumatism *arthritis*." Shelly's fists were clinched at her sides, a dangerous sign.

"Rheumatism *is* arthritis."

"No, it's not! Rheumatism is different than arthritis. When somebody's rheumatism is 'acting up' or when they're 'stove up' from bone pains, or feeling the weather in their bones, they deserve the respect and empathy due old age.

They don't want you to reach for your prescription pad and dash off 'Indocin' in undecipherable handwriting. Rheumatism is a symbol of the ponderous suffering of a long life, full of heartbreak, childbirth, hard work, death, and disappointment. Arthritis is an inflammation of the goddamn joints, which you may know how to treat, but you don't know shit about the other." Her chin pointed me.

"Why are you angry?" I got to my feet, extending my hands, palms up.

"I'm not angry. It just makes me mad when you go around with your superior notions that there's nothing wrong with the world that can't be quick-fixed by a careful application of advanced medical technology."

"You're not angry, but you're mad?" I smiled, realizing immediately that I shouldn't have said that and I shouldn't have smiled.

"I'm going to scream," she exclaimed. Tears welled in her eyes but hadn't overflowed. She was swallowing great gulps of air.

"Shelly, don't."

"I can't . . . talk intelligently . . . with you . . . . I . . ."

"Don't, Shelly, please!"

Shelly screamed. God, how she screamed. The garnitures on the mantel rattled. The urn with her father's ashes rattled, too.

"Shelly, tell me what's wrong. Is it PMS?"

Oh shit, I shouldn't have said that either. That one was right there in the rheumatism/arthritis dichotomy. But worse. A man, especially a doctor man, must never, *never* attribute female attitudes, moods, or philosophic observations to hormonal changes before or during menstruation or the pause activated by the cessation of said hormonal phenomena. Unless, of course, he is a gynecologist. Even a gynecologist must avoid with nimble dexterity words like *PMS, menstruation, moontime,* or *menopause,* especially if his patient is in the acute clutches of the syndrome he describes. He must, in short, hem and haw.

Shelly's second scream transcended the mere expression of anger and frustration. It was a timeless and archetypal female howl--a condemnation of general mankind, which had originated on the lisping tongue of the first Mother and had reverberated and amplified from the arbors of Eden down the ages through female blood. It was a cry that could stop any male in his tracks, because all male blood has coursed during its prenatal time in female veins and mingled with a mother's juices. It was a sound, like Hack's panther, to freeze-dry the blood:

"HAAAHiiiiiiiiiiEEEEEEEEEEEEEEEEEEEEEE!"

Now artesian water overflowed her eyes. "Put *that* in your damned notebook," she screeched, shaking her head and slinging tears. Shelly slammed the door, and the gold-framed photograph of her father fell. The photograph toppled the urn containing his ashes, but I caught the urn before it hit the floor, spilling only a pinch of Daddy, which I rubbed into the shag carpet with the toe of my white bucks. I stood on quaking knees, hugging the urn to my belly as the aftermath of Shelly's scream continued to buzz my vibrating brain.

"You've either been working too hard or you're a bigger damn fool than I thought," Hack had said when I fled to his house from Shelly's wrath.

Chapter Forty-Four

Y ou ever heard of Sisyphus?" Hack asked out of the blue. He was butchering an eight-point buck hamstrung on a gambrel hook he had hoisted with his truck. He'd been hunting. I sometimes went with him, sitting in the pre-dawn hours without a gun, watching the woods come alive, taking notes. I was going more now that Shelly was gone.

The deer had been flayed downward to the neck, and the hide was draped over the rack. Warm viscera lay in a bloody washtub, smoking in the cold January air. Hack's bare arms were bloodied to the elbow. He reached into the rib cage, expertly cutting the muscle inserts and removing the eight-inch tenderloins, putting them in a plastic baggy for my supper. Then he began slicing out the backstraps, the long muscles that ran along the spine from the shoulder to the haunch.

"Sure," I said after thinking over his question. "Sisyphus is the Titan condemned to push a heavy rock up a mountain. When he reaches the peak, the rock rolls back down. He's condemned to this meaningless task for eternity."

"Well, think of yourself as Sisyphus, and think of your hospital as the rock."

"What do you mean, Hack?"

"You been sandbagged from the word go." He tested the edge of his knife with the pad of his thumb. Before he had started, he'd shaved a spot on his forearm. The tarbrush hair on his arm was enough to dull a good hunting knife or a scalpel.

"How sandbagged?"

"You remember when you first got shanghaied aboard Trafford Hospital, when your car broke down and Melvin Dryden wouldn't fix it on credit? You had to work off the bill at the hospital. Well, we needed a doctor then. And the town council was bound and determined to have one besides Lee Bob Parker and that dopehead Flowers to help out Carl Hogue. So you happened along, and nobody wasn't inclined to turn you a-loose. Most everybody in town wanted Trafford to survive. With you on board and Hogue at the wheel, and with Benbow Hutchinson's promise of four million dollars, it looked like Trafford might float. But there was one somebody who didn't want Trafford to survive, and he still don't."

"Who?"

"You pretty good at figuring things out, so let's see how you can do on this one. What was the only glimmer of fiscal hope Trafford had when you landed here?"

"Like you just said, Benbow Hutchinson had promised to leave Trafford four million in his will."

"Who got that? Or, put another way, who kept Trafford from getting that right sizable chunk of change?"

"Denise Carswell Hutchinson, Benbow's child bride and junior of sixty years."

"That's right, but did you know Denise was a hooker from Phoenix City, Alabama, whose massage parlor was bankrolled by Karl Wright? Wright brought Denise to Grady, set her up, and sicked her on Benbow Hutchinson for the sole purpose of sinking Trafford."

"Why would he do that?"

"So *he* could buy it." Hack paused, scratching his nose with his rolled cuff, raising his bloody knife and forearm into the air.

"Of course," I said, "that's what he's been doing all over south Georgia. Health for profit, a good investment, big bucks."

"He expects to turn Trafford into a eye surgery center, a new division of Southern Vision for his nephew Dr. Country Trulane."

"How could you know that?"

"I ain't *suppose* to know that, so I'll be obliged you don't say nothing."

Then suddenly I knew. Beulah Wright Parker. Hack, despite his hatred of her family and his contempt for her husband, was still consorting with Beulah.

"Aw Hack," I said.

"What?" He cut away the shoulders and put them in plastic garbage bags. It amazed me that you could remove the shoulders without cutting bone. No bones, only muscle and ligaments, joined a deer's front shoulders to its body.

"Nothing, except I can't believe Country Trulane would be a part of a plot to bankrupt a hospital."

"He's not. He's just your typical booksmart doctor with his head up his ass. His Uncle Karl sends him to school and sets him up. Country ain't concerned with the business end of anything. Uncle Karl says, 'tell you what, boy. I'm gonna open up a new division of Southern Vision that will lock up the southern tier of the state and make you the medical director. You'll knock down a cool million. How's that?' 'Oh that's swell Uncle Karl. I'm only making $750,000. as it is. Who knows when I'll have to add another wing on the mansion?' Besides, Trulane's taking his services to people that need them, restoring the eyes of the blind. He's a good doctor, doing his job in a system that worships the buck."

"So that's why Country Trulane was such a good sport when he lost at stickbirds," I said, peeking around Hack into the chest cavity of the buck.

"He's a sport, all right." Hack decapitated the deer by slicing through the muscle around the neck and finding a spot between the vertebra with the long blade to sever the spinal cord. When he inserted the point of his knife and

206

twisted his wrist, the head came off with the hide attached. Hack lifted it by the horns and laid it in the bed of the pickup. The rack was deformed and uneven, the kind of deer Hack harvested. He believed in leaving the trophy bucks to improve the herd. He culled the young "scrubs," which were better to eat anyway.

"He didn't have no choice but to be a sport," Hack continued. "Paul Dudley and you stood there watching him lose fair and square. He better lay down and die before he welshes on a bet at Tailfeathers, but he put up a better scrap than I thought he would. I wasn't messing around. I was trying my dead level best to put him under from that first bird on, none of that bullshit about missing a few on purpose to sweeten the pot."

"No. Don't you see, he *had* to perform a cataract operation for the certificate of need," I said. "He had to do an eye operation at Trafford anyway, to have it on the records. He would have done it with or without a chance to win the disk. Otherwise he couldn't cite a precedent when he applied for the conversion to an outpatient surgery after the takeover."

Hack grinned. "You mean the hospital has to have already done what Wright wants to do in order to do it."

"Something like that." I thought about it for a moment. Then I said. "Hack, I know you probably betrayed a trust with Beulah by telling me about the takeover. I want you to know I'm touched by your loyalty to me and to the hospital."

"Well, I hate to admit it, but sometimes when a man's torn between the opposite wills of two equally esteemed acquaintances, he's got to consider the matter of right and wrong."

"I know it wasn't an easy decision."

"No, it wasn't. As you may already know, Beulah's got something going for her you ain't never had."

"What's that?"

"A vagina."

"In light of that, thanks again."

"Put those little tenderloins on ice and let them cool down for a day or they won't be fit to eat," he warned. "Here, take you a backstrap too. Cut it in steaks and put it on the grill."

"I've got to go to the office. I can put the tenderloins in the refrigerator there. Put the deer in *your* freezer. I don't cook much any more."

"You can put the backstrap in the refrigerator too. Slice it into little steaks about a inch and a half thick and freeze them in little portions you can cook up when you get through at the clinic."

"O.K. Thanks. Can you handle it from here?"

Hack grinned. "Gee, I think so."

Chapter Forty-Five

Speaking of Beulah Parker's vagina, Beulah came in for a pap smear and breast cancer screening examination the Tuesday following Shelly's spontaneous exodus. As a matter of office protocol, either Shelly or Nancy chaperoned gynecological procedures, but Shelly, of course, was gone and Nancy wasn't in yet, so I began the examination unattended. Early May, ebullient as always, was in position at the reception desk, assuring our patients of Jesus' love, brightening the corporeal and spiritual horizons of everybody.

"I sometimes wonder if perhaps they are too small," Beulah sighed. She was seated on the edge of the examination table, holding open her paper gown like an artificial butterfly. I thought absurdly of Mary Lou's proposed breast reduction. A Hollywood doctor could set Mary Lou and Beulah side-by-side and liposuck from one to the other, a transfusion.

"Raise your arms, please."

There were hairline scars around the areola of her nipples. Her breasts were precisely the size she'd ordered. They comprised as lovely a pair as ever adorned woman. With a detached manner, I had her lie down on the table. Standing above, I avoided her eyes and began palpating her breasts looking for masses. Both nipples erected. "Ummm," she said as I compressed each breast to demonstrate dimpling, "Ummm." I pressed the breasts against the chest wall with my fingertips, noting the presence of the turgid nipples. The paper crinkled as she shifted her hips. Then I had her sit up, hanging her legs over the edge of the table while I sat on the examining stool and had her raise her arms as I checked to make sure the hardened nipples were symmetrically placed and that their relative position was consistent. Beulah's breasts were perfectly symmetrical, abnormally so, since most women have a slightly larger left breast.

"My arms are getting tired, Doctor," she said. "May I rest my elbows on your shoulders?"

I tried to continue my clinical examination, but Beulah's breasts were too close for me to focus upon. That's not to say that they were too close to mesmerize me. My head swam, the tides of my brain coming under the gravitational influence of those sculpted orbs. "Hum," I said, which is what I say to sound professional.

"Are you finding anything?" her voice whispered above my bowed head.

"Uh no. Everything seems in good order." I turned my profile to the subjects of my examination, concentrating on the Eye Examination chart, when suddenly her arms wrapped around my neck. Something akin to a pencil eraser penetrated my ear while another fleshy intruder bobbled against my nose and mouth, threatening suffocation. Immediately there was a sharp rap at the door. "Nancy!"

I mumbled.

"That tickles," Beulah whispered. "Don't talk."

I gently pushed her chest away from my face, very gently. With Shelly gone my resistance to lust had weakened. "Ahem, we're a little too close. Let me, uh, move back just a little?" I wheeled around.

"Oh Nancy! Will you prepare a vaginal speculum for a pelvic examination, please!" My penlight palsied as I transilluminated her breasts, revealing some translucent silicone masses but no opacity or any other abnormalities.

"Right away, Doctor," Nancy called through the door. Preparing the stainless steel speculum meant submersing it in warm water to heat it up and lubricate it, making penetration of the vagina more easily executed and more comfortable for the patient.

I asked Beulah to lie back down on the table and to put her feet in the stirrups. "Burrr," she smiled, throwing the gown back from the lower half of her body, "your stirrups are icy." She wiggled her candy-apple toenails.

"Not yet," I said. "You can keep your gown closed until my assistant comes. The better to keep you warm." Nancy came in with the speculum and a pap smear brush.

"She's not going to stay in here with us, is she? I'd be embarrassed," Beulah said. "With my legs up like this, I feel so . . . vulnerable."

"Oh, don't worry about my sister Nancy. She's a professional."

"Yep," said Nancy. "Office protocol. I'll be here to make sure my big brother doesn't get too fresh or get in over his head."

I scowled sidelong at Nancy, put on a pair of rubber gloves, and sat inside the hospitable V of Beulah's legs. I inserted my index finger into her vagina, retracting the introitus posteriorly, then began inserting the closed blades of the speculum, but the instant the speculum entered her, her vagina contracted violently, like a snail that has encountered lemon juice, and her buttocks scooted up the table tearing the paper. "Yike!" she yipped. "Oh!"

"What's wrong?" I demanded, noticing that the handles of the speculum through my latex gloves were uncomfortably cool. I touched the blades, which were stinging cold. They sweated condensation. Beulah's heels were out of the stirrups, digging into the table, ripping paper as they pushed a puckered vagina out of harm's way.

"My God," I told Nancy, whose hands were planted on her hips, "this thing's like ice!"

In a second Beulah was up, casting off her gown and throwing on her clothes. "You're not ever putting another damned thing up me!" she said, storming out.

"Oatsie, what did she mean *another*?" Nancy raised an eyebrow.

"What do *you* mean, submersing my speculum in cold water?"

"I didn't," she said indignantly. "I put it in the freezer. I dipped the handle in warm water so your fingers wouldn't get cold."

"Why, for Christ's sake? Beulah Parker is just about the only patient we've got who can afford to pay her bill."

"I figured the hussy might need cooling off. And you too."

"It cooled her off," I admitted.

"Did you see her vapor breath, Doats?" Nancy laughed.

"I wasn't watching her mouth." I smiled. I'd never been able to stay mad at Nancy for very long. We were both quiet for a few moments before Nancy spoke again. "Shelly called," she said coyly.

"What? Where is she? When's she coming home?"

"She's not coming back. At least not anytime soon, but she told me to tell you hello."

"*Hello?*" I pulled off my latex gloves and tossed them.

"Well, that's what she said." Nancy pursed her lips. "She probably meant more, like 'I love you uncontrollably and irrevocably so that my heart fibrillates at the mere mention of your name, but you can kiss my cleft ass for storming Dixie like a Mongol, overrunning my hometown, abolishing my job and making it virtually impossible for critical patients to get anywhere near a Band-Aid without hitchhiking.' That's probably what she meant."

"Where is she?" I replaced the torn paper on the examination table.

"Vanderbilt."

"That's impossible. I've tried to reach her through the campus locator. They don't have her listed."

"I believe her," Nancy winked. "Don't you?"

"She actually enrolled in law school?"

"She had an appointment for spring semester. Didn't you know that?"

"I knew she did a long time ago, but she canceled out. I *thought* she canceled out."

"Why would she do that?"

"For me," I said, immediately revising. "For us. For Grady."

"She thinks she's done all she can do for Grady. Unless she specializes in malpractice and returns to spearhead a purge to rid the county of Yankee doctors."

"Give me her number, Nanny. I've got to call her," I begged.

"I don't have it, Oatsie. She knew if she gave it to me I'd have to give it to you. She said she'd call you sometime."

"*Sometime?* Well, why'd she leave?"

"She was out of work."

"She didn't need to work. She could have married me. I'd have taken care of her."

Nancy made a face like she had just stepped barefoot in pig shit. "YOOOOOOH, Otis! Shelly's not going to marry somebody who doesn't recognize the importance of her life's work."

"If her work is so important, why is she becoming a lawyer?"

"That work will be important too. She's going to bring a class action suit against the Wrights and The Lilies of the Field Nursing Home as soon as she passes the bar, and she's got some other good ideas."

"Why are you acting so smug?" I said, "Whose side are you on anyway?"

"Hers, Oatsie-Doats. Hers."

Chapter Forty-Six

"Oh, Dr. Stone!" Early May Culpepper gasped, "Hack Singletree had a massive coronary. Melvin Dryden had to pick him up with the wrecker at the Magnolia Motel and take him to the emergency room. Dr. Maloy is with him now."

"I think I know what he was doing at the Magnolia Motel, but why did Melvin bring him in?"

"Well, you know we ain't got a ambulance no more."

"I'm well aware of that, Miss Culpepper." Nobody in Grady missed the opportunity to point out that Grady no longer had an ambulance service and had to wait thirty minutes for the unit from Flint. And nobody felt the sting of that loss like I did.

"Well, some lady called 911, and the sheriff's office dispatched the wrecker since Rooster Bootman wasn't around. The wrecker's the only other vehicle's got a radio."

"Why didn't the lady bring him to the emergency room?"

"I don't know, Dr. Stone. She was gone by the time Melvin got there, and she wouldn't leave a name when she called in."

I knew why.

Beulah Parker's tan diesel Mercedes had rattled out of my office parking lot straight to the Magnolia Motel, where she had ordered out for something to take the chill off her visit to the doctor. Fornication was retribution for Beulah, and she went after it with a vengeance. After screwing Hack into a coronary, she didn't have the decency to show up at the hospital where she might be asked to account for her coincidental whereabouts. I couldn't see what difference that would make. Everybody in Grady, with the possible exception of Lee Bob Parker, knew about Hack and Beulah. It takes a special kind of woman, I thought, to crawl out from under a man turning blue from a massive myocardial infarction and abandon him. Sorry, but I've got an appointment at the hairdressers, she might as well have said. Just read the Gideon until somebody comes.

Maloy telephoned to tell me Hack was alive in the Trafford emergency room, but barely. "I think I've got him stabilized for the time being on a nitro drip, but he'd have been a lot better off if somebody could have gotten to him sooner. When he came in, he was in ventricle fibrillation. Melvin said he passed out about a minute before they pulled into the ER parking lot. We had to shock him back. We don't know if there's any brain damage. With Hack it's going to be hard to tell."

I knew Hack's condition was serious. Maloy wouldn't joke about brain damage unless the situation was grim. Generally upbeat and optimistic, Jim saved his dark humor for dark days.

Go ahead and say it, I thought. Hack's dying or disabled because you sacked Shelly and the other EMT's.

"There's no telling how much damage was done while he was flopping around on the Magic Fingers before Melvin got there," Maloy continued. "I'm having him transported to Putnam, where Mitchell Hoots and Jeff Roberts are on the lookout. Their ambulance is due in about 10 minutes."

"Is he conscious?"

"He's in and out. I've got him on morphine. He woke up once, looked Margaret Holt straight in the face, and asked her was it good for her too. Then he drifted off again."

"Stay with him. I'm coming to ride him in."

———

The Putnam EMT's were loading Hack up when I got there. I climbed in and saw him pale and sweaty, strapped into the stretcher with the clear plastic oxygen tubes nasally inserted. I took his hand as we headed out. It was cold, limp, and clammy as a slab of rough meat--like a dead rock bass. His system was clamping down, trying to sustain blood pressure. There's nothing that looks more helpless than a big man dropped by a heart attack, and I felt as helpless as he looked.

I wanted to ride with him to maintain a lidocaine and nitroglycerine drip, but really there was nothing I could do. His EKG indicated he'd had a large anterior injury. If the clot propagated and completely blocked his coronary artery--about the size of a pencil lead-- he'd go into irreversible cardiogenic shock and die. I just sat there watching his telemetry, praying that the PVC's wouldn't run together into fibrillation. I was ready with the paddles if they did, speeding down the Flint highway, swaying in a capsule of hysterical sirens with the grim cargo of a man, my friend, on the threshold of death. It was just a matter of luck whether the clot propagated or not.

Then one crusty eye opened, bloodshot and steady, like the eye of a goat that had been run over by a train. "You wouldn't happen to have a drink of shine on you, would you, Doc?"

I shook my head. "Your whisky drinking days are over."

"What if I just cut back to 100 proof? Just wean off the stump and go to drinking red whiskey like a gentleman." He stopped to catch his breath. "Which would represent a considerable reduction, don't you know?"

"You're through with red whiskey too."

His eye closed again. At least he was able to recognize me, to know I was with him. Maybe that was a comfort. Maybe not. He might have felt better if

Hartwell, the Vet, was aboard the ambulance. I asked Hack if he wanted me to swing by the animal hospital. "The only difference in a dog and a man," he said with his eyes still closed, "is a dog knows how to get his ass home on a rainy night."

After a long moment both eyes opened, startled at first, then calm. "Whew," he said. "Don't you know that Beulah Wright Parker's one dynamite piece of ass!"

"I wouldn't know about that."

"You will, you stay in Grady long enough. If you don't know first hand you can witness the aftermath of her destruction strapped to this here stretcher." He smiled weakly.

"She could have brought you in instead of calling the wrecker."

"She was protecting me." Hack's voice was tired.

"How so?"

"Old Lee Bob find out I was porking his wife, he'd take me off his Christmas card list." Hack closed his eyes and paused. "But I'd heap rather Lee Bob knew about the 'Magnolia Connection,' than Mary Lou."

"Don't worry about Mary Lou," I said.

"Well, if it should happen to come up in polite conversation, you can tell her I'm through with Beulah. A brilliant fellow like myself, he don't have to get used and left for dead more than once by the same gal to get the message."

"Hush," I said, "you rest now. How about some more morphine?"

"Naw," he said drifting off again. "I want me some *shine*."

Hack's PVC's were grim testimony to the severity of his injury and its resulting irritability, but he was hanging on, and there didn't seem to be a lot of brain damage, although, like Maloy said, on Hack brain damage might not be so easy to detect.

The twenty-five-mile trip to the Putnam Memorial was the longest trip I'd ever taken. I could almost feel the blood clot building as flotsam and jetsam of the restricted blood collected in the blocked artery. I didn't want to lose this renaissance redneck, who'd overcome his natural prejudice against Yankees and physicians to befriend and teach me the skills I needed for spiritual survival in the deep South.

I thought long and hard about the wisdom of sacrificing the ambulance for the hospital. How much of my determination to save Trafford at all costs was a result of my training to be an academic internist--AN INTERNIST IS NOTHING WITHOUT A HOSPITAL? Maloy, an internist himself, felt that Putnam Memorial could be convinced to accept our patients on a wholesale basis. He thought the time lost during the 25-mile ride to Putnam would be made up in most cases by well-trained EMTs, who could stabilize trauma victims better than

Trafford's ER anyway. He didn't feel that a hospital that couldn't handle farm accidents, gunshots, or childbirth was such an invaluable asset to a community like Grady. I saw Hack to the ICU. After he was cathed, I ran down Mitchell Hoots and Jeff Roberts.

"Proximal left anterior descending lesion, 90% block," said Hoots, the Emory trained cardiologist whose brilliance in his field was sometimes disguised by the illusion that he was peering amiably through a foggy windshield, "but he's got good function, so Roberts can bypass him."

"I'll cut first thing in the morning," Roberts said. "I don't want this fish to spoil."

"Mind if I scrub?"

Chapter Forty-Seven

Dr. Jeff Roberts, already four minutes late, stormed into the OR lounge bitching about his perfusionist. Roberts scheduled his first surgery in the predawn hours and was therefore referred to by anesthesiologists and scrub nurses as Doctor Frankenstein. He wore a Massey Ferguson baseball cap and had fingers yellowed to the second joint by nicotine stains. But Roberts wasn't the only one in the lounge. Jack Puckett Middlebrooks had agreed to do a charity D & C for me. Gordon Powell was removing a gall bladder. After Hack, Roberts was scheduled to by-pass another charity. Thursday was Socialist Day in the OR, they quipped. These patients couldn't pay a penny, but the doctors joked that they didn't need to make money since they were too busy to spend it on anything but malpractice insurance, and to their credit they provided the same standards of care for the indigent as for the affluent.

"Watch your piggies in there, Dr. Middlebrooks," Roberts warned. Three years before, a histerscope had dropped from a vagina during a D & C and had broken Puck's little toe. The other Putnam doctors hadn't let him live it down, insisting that the histerscope provided an epiphany for Middlebrooks that equaled Newton's apple.

"Let's hit the deck," Roberts ordered. Hack had said he wanted me to observe, since Henry Hartwell was busy spaying a cat. Roberts said sure. "*Bailamos*," he told his surgical team, "Let's us dance."

I spoke to Hack before Mark Moran, the anesthesiologist, put him under. Shrouded in a hospital gown and tranquilized by Valium, he lay supine on the operating table, flirting with the circulation nurse who'd heard every line that could come out of a human mouth.

"Dr. Moran, cool this old boy down, if you please," she said, her eyes twinkling. "Sweet dreams, Mr. Singletree."

Dr. Moran placed a mask over Hack's nose and mouth and tuned the IV until Hack's face sagged into unconsciousness. He looked like some strange depilated giant that had fallen from a beanstalk, goofy, the whites of his eyes showing until the nurse put ointment in them and taped them shut. His mouth turned up at the corners in an oddly angelic smile. Then the team inserted tubes and sensors in every orifice of his body, including some places that hadn't been orifices when Hack checked in. Two black orderlies held up his bald legs one at a time and painted them yellow with betadine. Then they stained his abdomen and his shaven genitals. Scrub nurse Kathy Loy, her latex clad hand glistening with KY jelly, stretched Hack's flaccid penis to insert the lubricated catheter. The orderlies slapped palms. "Whoooee," one said, "for a white man, that dude have a righteous hang!" Kathy, holding Hack's penis like a wilted flower, shot them

217

a glance that shortened their necks. Their shoulders protecting their ears, they grinned sheepishly and padded out.

Andy Lyons, Roberts' P.A., took a scalpel from its sterilized wrapper and sliced Hack from just above the instep to six-inches above the knee, removing a worm-colored saphenous vein. The betadine-tinted vi-drape made Hack's bald chest look like ham rind.

Roberts placed his index finger on Hack's solar plexus. With his right hand he touched the point of his scalpel at the top of the breast bone, and sliced the length of his chest. Flesh parted, the yellow fat beaded with sparse bright berries of blood. Roberts cauterized the tiny bleeders with his bovie. Then the Stryker saw, rattling like rocks in a tin can, halved Hack's chest so that it looked like something Hack himself would throw on a barbecue grill. Roberts turned the screws of the chest retractor and torqued open the rib cage. He opened the pericardium where lay Hack's generous heart. Coated with tallow, it squirmed and thumped like a snake in a bag.

Roberts removed the mammary artery. Vacillating between humming Simon and Garfunkle's "Sound of Silence" and quoting long passages of Keats, he barked amiable commands to the scrub nurse, anesthesiologist, and perfusionist. These strange and eclectic noises were punctuated by the soft slap of a forceps or clamp into his latex glove. "*When I have fears that I may cease to be* reverse scissors (slap)--*dah-dah-dah, dee-dee, dah-dah*--forceps (pop) *before my pen has glean'd my teeming brain--dee-dee, dah-dah, dee-dee-dee--dee-deee*, sponge." He attached one end of the saphenous vein to Hack's aorta.

There was an otherworldly ambience created by the blunt man who looked more like a diesel mechanic than a thoracic surgeon. He spliced Hack's vessels with prodigious dexterity of fingers that didn't seem to belong to the hairy, muscled forearms buried in Hack's chest. Dr. Moran monitored the patient as Roberts poured icy slush from an ordinary looking plastic pitcher into Hack's chest to still his heart.

In an irrelevant flash, I saw the OR as a recording studio. The perfusionist was seated behind the heart-lung machine with its clear plastic wheels turning like a gigantic tape player, pumping clear tubes of Hack's crimson juice, while Dr. Moran manned the anesthetic machine and resuscitator with its monitors and its bellows pumping like a slow musical piston. At that moment the scrotal rubber bulb of the manual resuscitator seemed obscurely attached to a hidden horn, which I imagined would honk or beep when squeezed. Moran reached like a drummer to IV's, tubes, and settings. Kathy and the other nurses in provocative masks that emphasized resplendent eyes fanned mortal melodies with hand and wrist, gliding around the OR in sterile booties. Roberts, elbow deep in the cavern of Hack's thorax, orchestrated life into the cadaverous form spread open at the center of the group, humming, singing, quoting poetry as he conducted.

I could see the red tattoo of ruptured capillaries along the left side of Hack's heart as though someone had sprinkled it with paprika. "There's what he did jumping that broad's bones in the Magnolia Motel," Roberts said, "making the beast with two backs."

"He says he's learned the lesson of his wayward ways."

"To hell with that," said Roberts. "I'm gonna fix him up so he can really misbehave."

Using Hack's mammary artery and the saphenous vein, Roberts skillfully bypassed the occluded areas, four of them, splicing blood vessels into cardiac muscle with sutures the size of kitten claws. When he finished, he stepped back and bowed individually to every member of his team, who bowed back.

"Let's kickstart this big fellow," he said. "Hand me the paddles." Roberts' surgical gown looked like a butcher's smock. "Contact!--da-da, dee-dee, dah-dah-dah-daaah! '. . . Till love and fame to nothingness do sink . . . .'" Hack's heart hit two licks and stopped. Roberts looked down his nose. "Humm, do you reckon this fellow knows how to put an overworked surgeon on a bigmouth bass?"

"I can warrant and guarantee it," I said. "There's not a better man for that in the whole state. You also just swapped for the fishing rights at Loonie Lake."

"Let's hit him again." The paddles against Hack's heart juiced it and made it kick and flop.

"There he goes," Kathy said.

Finishing, Roberts said: "Well, close him up Andy. Otis, let's you and me go talk to his girl Mary Lou and eat some lunch before we do your charity case. I never throw away four thousand dollars on an empty stomach."

We left Andy lacing up Hack's sternum with stainless steel wire. We put lab coats over our scrubs and went to the OR waiting room to tell Mary Lou that the surgery was over and the patient was alive, well, and repentant.

Chapter Forty-Eight

The late winter rain had announced itself with an easterly wind, blowing the leaves underside up and white, sucking wet air from the Gulf of Mexico. A fly's loud fumbling buzz at the window, the smoke from chimneys lying low to the ground: Hack had taught me to watch these things to predict rain, to know when a front was coming through.

I stood in my kitchen, watching last night's open bottle of Club soda resume its fizz. Low barometric pressure. The deer will be moving now, I thought. If I hunted, now would be a good time to kill a deer. I knew I was thinking what Hack was thinking from his hospital bed in Flint. The last time I'd visited him, he'd been prowling the halls with a walker, encumbered by telemetry, as cheerful nurses monitored his EKG and vital signs at the nursing station. They said they could tell when he was *trash*ing. A hound is said to *trash* when it trails some animal other than a coon. A bird dog is said to be trashing when it points a shitbird, which is a non-game bird that to an inexperienced dog smells like a quail.

The rain had started in a slow drizzle when the telephone, turned down to a rattle, brought me back from my bone-gnawing longing for Shelly. It was Rooster Bootman.

"Doc, there's a wreck on 85. I'll pick you up on the way out there."

I hardly had time to get my jacket before Clarice howled--Awroooo, awroooow--followed by Rooster's siren. Shelly had left Clarice at Hack's house with a note asking him to keep her with his dogs. I was a little surprised by Shelly's willingness to entrust Clarice to him, although she couldn't help being somewhat moved by Hack's unswerving loyalty to my cause. Tension relaxed even more when the Maloys came on the scene and all but dissolved with Mary Lou's appearance, but apparently Clarice wasn't so easily converted. She promptly ran away from Hack's kennels and came to Lake Loonie, where her mournful eyes reflected my loneliness and loss. Maybe Clarice's patronage at my house was a good sign, foreshadowing Shelly's eventual and prodigal return. I walked out to the porch and saw Rooster's patrol car bucking down the dirt road, flashing blue.

"Where's yore bag?" Rooster shouted, reaching over to open my door. I tossed in my gas mask pack.

"Where've you been, Rooster? Doctors don't carry bags anymore. Or make house calls."

"Sure, let's go!"

The rain was heavier now. Rooster's windshield wiper knocked out a dull rhythm as we sped down my long driveway, slinging mud.

"Who is it? Do you know who it is?" I became suddenly aware that I had been here long enough for Grady to become my community. I realized that the odds were pretty good that I'd be acquainted with whoever was involved in the accident. There was more than an outside chance that somebody involved had visited my office with one of the numerous ills that plagued the county population.

"Well, one of the Wright boys or both of them is in it," Rooster said, "and there's another car with two black women, I don't know who. One car must've rear-ended the other one."

"How many are hurt?"

"I think all of them's banged up some, but there's a old lady must be hurt pretty bad. They ain't got her out the car yet. It's out in front of Bucky Cloud's place. He's the one called it in."

When we topped the last hill before the Clouds', I could see the cars and the people standing around. Bucky, a pecan farmer, was barefoot in the yard, while his wife stood on the front porch, hugging her shoulders. A red car I recognized as Wilkin Wright's was sideways in the highway with a bashed-in grill and a spider-web windshield, while the other car, an old purple Buick with a demolished trunk, was nosed into the ditch.

A young black girl was in turns running to the Buick and back to the highway, where she danced in hysterical circles in the rain, pulling her plaited hair with her fists. When we were close enough, I recognized Miss Ethel Hargrove's great granddaughter Cyrilla.

"It's Big Mamma! It's Big Mamma!" she cried, running up to the patrol car as the siren was winding down. "She's bleeding and I cain stop the blood."

"Cyrilla!" I shouted.

I waded down the ditch to the passenger side of the Buick. I saw Wilkin jump out of the Mustang and limp up to Rooster Bootman.

"Those niggers just pulled right out in the road!" he shouted. "Ask Marvin if they didn't."

"I don't see no place they could've pulled out from," said Rooster Bootman. Marvin was standing in the Clouds' open carport, his head back, holding a bloody towel to his forehead.

The current of muddy water tugged at my ankles. Cyrilla was behind me, "I cain stop the blood! I cain stop the blood!" she cried.

You're a doctor, so cool it, I kept telling myself, wondering why I felt so helpless, wondering why my knees were weak and I had to keep trying to swallow my swollen heart. The car door fell from its hinges into the ditch when I opened it. Miss Ethel sat erect, her right hand wrapped in a monogrammed towel. "Miss Ethel, what have you done to yourself now?" I said, feigning composure with a cracked voice.

She smiled vaguely. "Hello young doctor," she said. "I'm afraid I done gone too far this time. Just look here what a mess I has made of Mrs. Cloud's good face towel." The towels and lap of her house dress were saturated with blood-- blood nearly devoid of clotting factor, thinned by Coumadin I had prescribed. But then I saw the hematoma, a great, ugly swelling the size of a football on the old woman's hip. There was internal bleeding too. On that prescription pad, I now realized, I'd scribbled out the death warrant of the oldest woman in Grady county. I had sealed it by my vote to discontinue the ambulance service in favor of continuing a bankrupt hospital. Good money after bad.

"Call my daddy!" Wilkin yelled to Mrs. Cloud. "Tell him to come get me. I'm hurt! Tell him some niggers pulled out in a old Buick!"

"Shut up, boy, and put your hands behind your back," said Rooster. "You open up your mouth again, I moan stomp a mud hole in your ass."

Bucky Cloud came over, soaking wet. "I got a camper," he said. "I would've took her in, but I was scared to move her."

"We better use the patrol car so we can keep her warm," I said. "Will you get me a blanket, Bucky? Rooster, drive your car as close as you can get over here." Suddenly, absurdly, it occurred to me why Sheriff Bootman was called Rooster. In the rain his red hair stood up in a comb as he highstepped with jerky gallinaceous movements to his car.

I placed a rolled bandage against the pressure point on the inside of Miss Ethel's upper arm and wrapped it in gauze. The cut on the back of her hand still seeped blood. In other circumstances the wound would not have been serious. Ordinary blood would have clotted. Mrs. Cloud must have thought her best towels would make the best bandages too. I asked Bucky to bring a straight back chair.

As Rooster backed the patrol car across the Cloud's lawn, Mrs. Cloud ran out in the rain with a patchwork quilt. "Oh, Aunt Ethel," she said, "are you awright?"

"I be all right, honey," Ethel said softly. "Don't you worry, but that too nice a patch to mess up in all this blood."

"It's the nicest thing I got," bawled Mrs. Cloud. "You sewed it for mamma when I was a little girl."

"So I did," Miss Ethel smiled. "I do remember that patch."

I wrapped the quilt around her shoulders, and Rooster, Bucky Cloud, and I slid her into the chair and carried her across the ditch. She was not a small woman, but she was surprisingly light. I stepped on the car door in the running water and it shifted under my feet. When I looked down and saw the stream running red with Georgia clay, it seemed to me the entire earth was gashed open, bleeding beyond its capacity to replenish itself. I had never in my life felt so helpless, not even in the ambulance with Hack. I thought I'd feel helpless for the rest of my life.

We put Miss Ethel in the back seat between Cyrilla and me. She was shivering. She was dying. We both held her, trying to apply pressure to the places she was bleeding, trying to hold back the blood. We held her tightly, feeling her shiver, shivering ourselves.

Rooster was handcuffing Wilkin to the bumper of the Buick.

"Take me with you," Wilkin begged. "You know my daddy. You know who my daddy is?"

"Yeah, I know your goddamn daddy," said Rooster. "That's why I figure you too good to ride in the same car with these folks. Maybe you'll be sober by the time I get around to coming back, you and your brother."

"Handcuff me to the steering wheel then," Wilkin begged. "You can't leave me out in the rain."

"Please don't leave that child in the weather like that, Sheriff Bootman," said Ethel, her voice ebbing low. "Bring him on in the *po*lice car, and bring the other one on too."

I don't know if Rooster took Wilkin and Marvin to town to grant a dying woman's last request or whether he took them because I reminded him that he might prejudice his case by police brutality. But he took them, handcuffing Marvin to Wilkin and pushing them roughly into the front seat.

"I ain't done nothing," protested Marvin, whose facial lacerations had bled upon his shirt front and shoulders so that it looked like he was wearing a collar of red lace.

"Shut up," said Rooster, "you a accessory."

Later, I tried to remember if Miss Ethel's plea for Wilkin and Marvin constituted her last words. But I think she said one other word before she died. I'm not sure because I've relived her death in my dreams, and I can't distinguish clearly between imagination and reality. I think she uttered one word more as Rooster sped to Trafford, his siren screaming, moaning, then screaming again. "Glory," she said as her body fatally softened in my arms and in Cyrilla's.

"Gory?" I asked Cyrilla.

"Glory," said Cyrilla. "She say *glory*."

———————

We took Miss Ethel's body into the emergency room on a stretcher and waited for Rooster to deposit his prisoners and return to take us home. Margaret Holt wrapped us in hospital blankets. Cyrilla was calm now. Both of us were soaked in rainwater and her great grandmother's blood. "Will you be all right?"

I asked her. We hugged, holding tightly to each other for a long time, listening to rain, and I irrationally heaped yet another charge upon my self-incrimination. Besides the Coumadin and the ambulance, I was guilty of Miss Ethel's death by saving that little son-of-a-bitch Wilkin's life twice.

Rooster took Cyrilla home first, then drove me to Lake Loonie. On the way we passed Melvin Dryden's wrecker leaving the shop. It was on the way out to Highway 85 to tow in two abandoned cars. When we got to my house I invited Rooster in. "You want a drink of Hack's stump? I'm having one."

"No, much obliged," he said. "I reckon I'll get on back. That wharf rat Willetts's bound to be downtown by now with some writ demanding that I release them scumbags on account of they're so prominent."

"Why are you holding Marvin?"

"Possession. I found some weed in the little shitass' sock."

"That all?"

"Well Doc, I didn't have much time, did I? We'll go over the car soon as Melvin brings it in, maybe find some crack or snort."

"I'd like to see Wilkin put away."

"I'd like to see him go to the electric chair, but he'll get off. He'll always get off."

Holding my nose, I tossed down four ounces of Hack's moonshine. Then I took off my bloody clothes and soaked in the bathtub to remove the chill I'd gotten from the cold rain. I cried and called myself hideous names and telephoned directory assistance in Nashville to have the recording of a snotty operator tell me for the umpteenth time that Shelly's number was unpublished. Just like her address was *unknown*.

I drank some more of Hack's stump and made a momentous decision. I made up my mind I was going to Toa Plantation first thing in the morning and ask Lynwood Honer to talk to his boss, Robert McCormick Jones, about donating a new ambulance to the Grady County EMT service, which I was getting ready to do my dead level best to have reinstated. I'd beg if I had to. I'd ask Commissioner Worthy and Miss Ida to influence the County to dump the hospital, sell it to Wright, and use the increased revenue to fund a really first class ambulance service. We'd also soup up the health department, adding prenatal care and hypertension and diabetes programs. How ironic that I wanted to serve Wright's interests after fighting him for so long.

Then I got sick and threw up until I thought my eyes were going to pop. The moonshine made me so sick I thought death would come as a blessing, but when I went to bed, I knew where I was going next and what I was going to do. There's something about gazing into the vortex of a flushed toilet that brings a man to himself.

Chapter Forty-Nine

I called Melvin Dryden early the next morning to get him to bring me the Falcon so I could drive over to Toa. "Uh, I'll come at you," Melvin said. "You can run me back to the shop."

He arrived in Hack's green pickup truck. "It needs running," he explained, "to keep the battery up."

"Why don't you put the battery on a trickle charge and give me back my car?"

"All kinds of things starts going wrong with a truck that ain't drove," he continued. "The clutch plate sticks, the carburetor gums up, the tires rot. Besides, I got some finishing touches to do on the Falcon."

"What do you mean *finishing touches*? All you were supposed to do was grease it and change the oil. I left it overnight."

"Well Doc, I found a few other little things need doing, that's all. Ain't you overreacting some over a car that's old enough to vote?"

"Maybe I am," I admitted. "But since the first day I pulled into this town I've had automotive trouble of one sort or another, and every time I've taken my car to you to have it fixed, I've ended up with more trouble than I had before I came. If I'm overreacting it's because I've developed a healthy paranoia. I am, in the vernacular, a bitten dog."

"A *bit* dog, Doc."

"What?"

"It's a *bit* dog. The saying's 'It's the bit dog that hollers.'"

"This bit dog knows where he's going."

"You got *that* right!" Melvin was puzzled, but willing to agree to anything I said. I knew damned well he was hiding something.

"Dog get bit once, he'll stay *off* that trail, won't he, Doc?" He stopped the truck on the side of the road in front of his garage. Leaving the engine running, he opened the door to hop out. Miss Ethel's purple Buick sent a chill into my bone marrow.

"Pull in," I said.

"What for?"

"I want to see if my car is really in there."

"It's in there, I swear to God." He parked and stared through the windshield at the corrugated metal wall. "Doc," he began, "have you ever had a patient who came in for a check-up or maybe a cold? And after you looked them over some, they tested out with cancer or heart trouble or a ulcer."

I jerked the truck door open, swinging out and marching to the garage. "I want to see my car!" I shouted.

"Whoa Doc," said Melvin running after me. "Let me explain something to you."

The Falcon was inside the garage all right, I guess all of it was. The problem was the whole Falcon wasn't all in the same place. It was--to a degree I could not determine in a glance--disassembled. Both doors, the hood, and the right front fender had been removed. The engine, which hung suspended over the motor well on a chain horse, was also partially dismantled. The carburetor, separated from the air cleaner, lay on the floor surrounded by satellites of tiny screws, springs, and butterfly valves. A rectangular valve cover and its gasket lay on the stained, concrete floor, and the valves themselves along with their rocker arms were arranged in demented order around a hubcap, which nested six chrome lug nuts. The entire front seat had been removed, and the instrument panel hung from the dash by red, green, and white electrical wires. Somebody had performed exploratory surgery on my automobile.

"Who . . . how . . . what the hell!" I shouted. "What's happened to my car! God damn you, Melvin."

"Now hold on, Doc. Ain't none of this my fault, and you're overreacting. We ain't talking about no Lambergini. All you got in this car is a chicken. I never thought I'd see the day you'd cuss me like that over a chicken."

"I've got twelve hundred dollars worth of unpaid medical bills in that pile of disassembled shit. Melvin, why did you do this to me?"

"Me? Doc, I didn't have nothing to do with this. Mr. Singletree, Hack's old daddy, he done this here," Melvin said, stepping backwards.

"Melvin," I whispered, stalking him, "why did you leave Mr. Singletree unattended in your garage with my car?"

"I didn't. It was raining and cold. I couldn't leave him in the electric fence. I brought him down here and locked him in the office. I didn't figure I'd be gone long, but I had to move Wilkin's car first cause it was in the road and the sheriff wanted it compounded for evidence, so it was near about five hours before I could get back here. I forgot about the screwdriver in my desk drawer."

I lost control. I was bouncing up and down from a half squat, pointing to my engine hanging from its net of chains. I screamed: "Mr. Singletree didn't do THAT with a goddamn screwdriver!"

"Nosir, he took the door hinges off with the screwdriver. That's how he got in the garage and found the air wrench." Melvin shook his head, staring away and smiling a lopsided grin. "It's amazing what that old fart can do with a air wrench and a full set of sockets. If I'd had one more wreck last night to tend to, there's no telling what he could've done. He was fixing to pull your rear end when I brought in Miss Ethel's Buick."

There was an eerie ambience about the situation and the world in general that morning since I woke up still hung over from the residual effects of Hack's rot gut whiskey. On my way to ask an ecologist to beg an ambulance from a soft drink magnate, I discover that my car has been disassembled by the deranged father of the junior high principal, a patient of mine convalescing from a heart attack. I somehow never lose sight of my overall mission, which is to scuttle a hospital and bring home my lover, an ambulance driver currently attending first year law school at Vanderbilt. And I am disoriented, guilt ridden, and brokenhearted over the death of a one-hundred-year-old woman. I am also pissed off as a dirt dauber in a flash flood by a twenty-five-year-old junkie.

The front passed through, and the cold west wind swept the scud from the blue sky.

"You're in luck," Lynwood Honer said. "Mr. Mack is down with some friends quail hunting, finishing up the season. We can meet him for lunch at the Tsallahatchee Baptist Church. You can sue him for your boon over fried chicken."

"I don't want to interrupt his hunt," I said.

"You won't, but if he invites you to ride along, go. That'll mean he's seriously considering your proposal, maybe even decided to buy you another ambulance."

"He already knows what I want?"

"Yeah, I told him. I did you a favor. He doesn't like surprises."

My best hope lay in the fact that the Ecological Research Center had non-profit status and was therefore tax exempt. Mr. Mack didn't want to negatively impact the area by causing a loss in tax revenue, so he'd been considering grants to the county that would make up for it.

"Health care," Lynwood continued, "has been a pet project for Mr. Mack since he started coming here as a young man to hunt in the mid 1930's, when he bought quinine and paid nurses to distribute it to fight malaria. I wouldn't be surprised if your new clinic found a friend in Mr. Mack."

We entered a little backwoods church nearly identical to the one where Hack and I had attended George Hawkins' funeral. Lynwood led me to Mr. Mack, who introduced me to five other men. These were wealthy businessmen who had just stepped out of Abercrombie and Fitch. Mr. Mack, a lean wind-burnished man, was dressed in tattered canvas clothing and fine briar-bitten boots. I'd have made him out to be a hunting guide rather than one of the richest men in the state. He handed me a chicken box and ushered me with a gaunt hand on my shoulder. I sat down at a rough hewn table set up near the altar. He poured large glasses of sweetened iced tea and served them himself. I listened as the men talked about the weather, the wind, and the dampness of the wiregrass after last night's storm, and the dog's ability to smell. They planned the afternoon hunt--which coveys they would shoot in order to end up at the Big House by dusk for drinks and supper, and finally Mr. Mack invited me to join them. "Will you ride, or do you prefer the wagon?"

"The, uh, wagon."

"Should you change your mind, I or one of my saddle-sore guests will be glad to swap places."

The wagon, pulled by matched brown mules, was equipped with rubber tires, dog cages, and vinyl upholstery. Mr. Mack tied his chestnut behind and climbed up beside me as the other hunters passed, posting awkwardly, the leather of their fine English saddles creaking.

"Put Bear and Pattie down," Jones told the dog handler. "I want Dr. Stone to see a paradigm by which to judge all others."

Both dogs hit the ground running, but they, especially the solidly muscled liverspot pointer, seemed more intent on defecation than hunting quail. He stopped every ten yards, hunching into a trembling squat and looking around guiltily. "That's common in bird dogs," Mr. Mack explained. "The excitement and adrenaline of the hunt loosens their bowels. They'll get rolling in a moment."

"Neurogenic diarrhea," I said.

The mules plodded along, their rabbit ears flopping, and the wagon rocked as the wheels plumbed holes. The dogs galloped ahead through the wiregrass and longleaf pines, Bear ranging long, while Pattie, a svelte English setter, worked closely and carefully near the trainer, a lean man the color of Swiss chocolate. He sat straight in his U.S. Army saddle, blasting coded messages with his whistle. "Ho!" he called to the bouncing dogs. Then soon he shouted, "Point!" Our driver shook the reins, and both of the mules leaned vigorously against their harness. One broke wind.

Bear was frozen into rigor mortis at the edge of a bicolor patch, crouched forepaw raised, tail rigidly bowed. Pattie moved in behind him, honoring the point, herself in a softer but no less serious stance. "Pah tee, care fulll!" the handler called.

"Will you shoot?" my host invited.

"I'm a novice," I admitted.

Jones nodded, reaching up to a horseman, who removed an over and under shotgun from a leather scabbard and handed it down. Jones loaded the gun, showing me the safety, instructing me to walk with him into the covey rise. "Choose one bird," he said. "If you drop that one, single out another."

We walked carefully to the pointed dogs. Bear was locked so tightly into his point that every fiber in his body was taut as fiddle frets. I imagined I could hear the electric hum of his rigid muscles. His tail was tipped with red, bloodied by briars. It was a moment of charged excitement, of perfect quiet. I could feel my heart thumping in my throat. But obviously there were no birds on the ground before Bear's concentrated rattlesnake eyes. If there were, I would be able to see them.

Then suddenly the earth opened and the air exploded with loud rattles and blurred brown missiles. One bird came toward me, narrowly missing my head then sailing over the other hunters. The main body of birds came up in a whirlwind, flipping on their afterburners and sailing away before I nicked my safety off. Mr. Mack dropped two birds--*POAH, POAH*--while I stood dumbfounded with gaping mouth, watching two birds that looked like they'd been propelled by stretched rubber bands zing low to the ground over the next hill. By the time I got my safety off, it was over. Except for one bird, known to quail hunters as the *lingerer*, whose ploy it is to wait until after his comrades have left, after the dogs have broken point, and after the guns are empty. Then, taking his own sweet time, he hurls himself into the air, levels off, shits a visible white drop, then flies leisurely and contemptuously away.

I was never quite sure how I did it, but I killed that bird. Perhaps it would be more accurate to say that a stray pellet forced the bird to light sooner than he'd planned and Bear caught and retrieved it. To my credit, the shotgun was actually shouldered when it discharged in the general direction of the bob white, but I had shouldered purely for the propriety of not being caught standing there stupidly at port arms after the covey had flown. The gun went off more or less accidentally when the butt touched my shoulder.

"Fine shot, Doctor," said Mr. Mack, slapping me across the back. The other hunters applauded politely. "And you showed admirable discretion in your restraint," he said smiling.

"Restraint?"

"Yes, shooting the first bird, the one that flew over your head, would've endangered the men on horseback. The main body of the covey, except for two low birds, got up in front of me. I wouldn't have blamed you for blasting away at them, but the fact that you didn't showed good field manners. Of course, you couldn't shoot the low birds for fear of hitting the dogs, so you waited on the lingerer and made an admirable shot."

"Those birds scared me so badly I thought I was going to have neurogenic diarrhea," I said. The shotgun blast had reactivated my hangover. I felt like Hack's daddy had gone in after my brains with the air wrench.

"Well, did you enjoy it?"

"As a Southern lady friend named Mary Lou is fond of saying, 'It's as much fun as you can have with your clothes on.'"

"You'd be suspect if you didn't like it," said Mr. Mack. "By the way, you'll get your ambulance."

"When did you decide that?"

"I've been watching you rather closely since you appeared in Grady, and I find you to be an idealistic if somewhat impractical young man. I think it's admirable that you are trying to provide quality health care in an underserved area, and I decided to give you an ambulance last night, before you called to ask for one. There are provisions: one, you must purchase a new, fully equipped Ford chassis from the dealer whose name my secretary will provide. It will be fully equipped with the most modern technology available. How much will that cost?"

"Maybe $75,000."

"Well, I don't care what it costs so long as it's the best one available, the top of the line, but my auditors will need an itemized cost breakdown and invoice. Get it geared to handle dirt roads and muddy terrains, and make sure it has a cooler for amputated appendages and snakebite anti-venin. The final provision is this ambulance is to be donated anonymously in the memory of Miss Ethel Hargrove, my old friend who died last night on the way to the hospital." So that was it. The mention of Miss Ethel brought a lump, and I nodded, afraid to try my voice.

"Don't skimp," he warned. And I nodded again.

Chapter Fifty

J ack Puckett Middlebrooks volunteered to fly me to Nashville, where I was
to pick up the new ambulance and, I hoped, Shelly, who didn't know I was
coming. I'd sworn never again to brave the element of air with Puck
Middlebrooks, but when a man has been deprived of sleep, love, and wholesome
food for long sequential periods, he's not really himself. Besides, Puck promised
to resist the temptation for aerial acrobatics. "Not even a pedestrian loop-tee-lie,"
he swore, making a tri-fingered Boy Scout honor signal, which he converted to
"bird" for the runway assistant who forewarned catastrophe by peeking through
spread fingers as soon as he saw Middlebrooks walking towards an airplane.

Off the ground and into the flight pattern, Puck played devil's advocate,
preparing me for the resistance I'd encounter at Putnam Memorial when I
requested hospital privileges for myself, Maloy, and the new staff we'd recruited
in Atlanta at the National Health Corps conference. "You Commies want us to
encumber our hospital with the same problem that bankrupted yours," he shouted
over the engine, "the tired, poor, huddled masses--the indigent burden. You're
bringing in government doctors, representing socialized medicine, and you want
us to receive them with open arms and give them blanket approval without even
screening them."

He handed me a set of earphones and switched us to intercom. "Government
doctors are eight-to-fivers. When the five o'clock whistle blows, they'll go back
to Grady and leave us with after-hours emergencies and follow up."

"We won't do that," I said. "We're conscientious physicians, with the same
training and ethics you have."

"By the way, we have a statute that says our doctors must live within twenty-
five miles of the hospital so that they can respond in a timely manner to
emergencies. Grady is twenty-six miles from Flint."

The statute was to safeguard Putnam against itinerant surgeons. I had an
answer to that objection at least. Lake Loonie was exactly twenty-three miles
from Putnam. I'd measured the distance when Shelly warned me about the
statue. "The new staff will be board certified," I said, "and they've been trained
in major academic centers--Ohio State, Duke, Cornell, Tufts, Emory, and the
Medical College of Georgia. There shouldn't be any objections to their
credentials."

"There'll be some objections to your PA's. We've got enough *play* doctors
as it is with chiropractors and podiatrists."

"P.A.s are going to revolutionize rural medicine, streamline it. I can hire a
good P.A. for half what I'd have to pay a physician. They're going to make that
quality, availability, continuity we talk about possible. The real question in the

future of medicine is going to be: is quality health care a right or a privilege? If it's a right, citizens can't be denied access. You can't have babies being born in hospital parking lots just because the mothers don't have health insurance."

"Too many indigent patients will lower my profits so I can't pay my malpractice insurance," Puck said, "which for this one little doctor is over $50,000 a year. If you want to free me to take on more charity work, you'll have to follow Shakespeare's recommendation and kill all the lawyers. I've got to make a big profit to survive. So does Putnam Memorial, whose charter, by the way, calls for an open door policy. Of course even now we're starting to lose money, which is one good reason in favor of Karl Wright's plan for a hostile takeover of Putnam to make it a for-profit health care facility."

"Puckett, why did you choose medicine in the first place?"

"To serve humankind, for economic stability, and to have funnnn!" He pitched the Cessna into a nose dive that pressed my stomach into my sinuses. The patchwork earth expanded in the windshield.

"Stop, goddammit! You promiiiisssed!"

He leveled off, and soon we were in a landing pattern over Nashville.

Chapter Fifty-One

Puck rented a car and took me to the First Response Emergency Vehicle Manufacturing Company to pick up Grady County's new ambulance, which was a thing of beauty, brightly painted white with red letters spelling AMBULANCE backwards across the front. There was a blue six-point star of life with a one-snake caduceus in the center and the numbers 911 on the side. The snake seemed to be smiling seductively, licking the air. "Tell Shelly I said hello," Middlebrooks said with a cherubic smile.

"What?"

"Good luck!" he said.

I found a U-haul trailer and had the vendor hook it up to the rear bumper of the ambulance. Then I drove to Vanderbilt Law School on the prowl, waiting in parking lots, driving around buildings, cruising the cafeterias, buttonholing students and professors.

Finally I spotted her, crossing the campus in front of the administration building with a middle-aged man with an umbrella and a green three-piece suit. He had a graying mane and a leonine face like F. Lee Bailey. I cranked up the ambulance, turned on the bars of red and white flashing lights, and with the siren blasting, I jumped the curb and sped out across the lawn to save Shelly from her would-be mentor. My spinning dual wheels slung divots against the bouncing trailer. Student pedestrians scattered, dropping papers and books. "MOVE OUT OF THE WAY--MOVE OUT OF THE WAY," my voice broadcast from two 100-watt speakers of the juicy PA system. WHOOP, WHOOP, WHUP, ERRRRRRIIIINNNGGG. Boy what a siren! This one could frizzle hair. The siren backed down, and the ambulance bucked, bearing down on its two victims, who stood frozen in shock, blasted by the realization that the wild ambulance had singled them out to run down or terrify.

I slammed on the brakes, gouging wide ruts in the manicured lawn, swinging out of the door, charging Shelly. Shelly's professorial companion stepped back, red faced and bewildered.

She recognized me and started laughing. "Excuse me," I said to her companion. I took her into my arms, dipping her and kissing her passionately. Then I led her around the ambulance.

"Fully equipped and fast as a scalded cat, 140 mph," I said, opening the back door and bowing at the waist with a flourish that invited Shelly to enter. "Fast as a striped-ass ape," I continued, noticing a belly slightly more protuberant than it should have been. She stepped on the tongue of the U-Haul and entered the back of the ambulance. I had just opened the double doors of enchantment--an EKG monitor/defibrillator, a Life Pack 5, plush vinyl bench and matching captain's chair.

"It's beautiful," she said, trying out the captain's chair, touching the Thumper heart-lung resuscitator with her fingertips, shamelessly fondling the clear rubber hoses of the suction unit.

With exaggerated flourish I pulled the handle of the one-man gurney, which slid out the back upon the lawn, the wheels dropping automatically. Shelly's mouth fell open. She was snowed, and I knew it. She'd have thrown a fur coat in my face for participating in cruelty to animals. A $75,000 European sedan wouldn't have impressed her one iota. But an ambulance, well . . . everybody has their price. Shelly's was an ambulance with a 100% modular body with aluminum diamond-plated running boards and rub rails.

"What's going on here?" said the professorial asshole in the three-piece suit. The dispersed students reconverged, looking for gore.

"You're pregnant!" I said. "About five months!"

"Good diagnosis, Otis," Shelly said, sitting on the squad bench and patting it like a bed. "We might make a doctor out of you yet."

"Get in!" I ordered.

"I am in."

"Get in the front!" I led her around to the passenger's side and opened the door.

"See here!" said the Bailey clone, brandishing his umbrella. "I demand an explanation!"

"The dean of the law school ordered this ambulance to make a campus appearance to help Vanderbilt law students identify early on what they'll be chasing for the rest of their lives."

"I AM the dean of the law school."

"Well then," I said. "how do you want me to bill you for the emergency vehicle demonstration?"

We sped away, sounding the 200-watt multitone siren--wail, high-low, air-horn, and yelp--circling the administration building once for good measure, showing off our 4-10 positive traction rear end.

"What's the U-Haul for?" she asked.

"I'm taking you home. We're going back to Grady. Clarice misses you."

"I don't have a place to live."

"Yes, you do," I said, reaching behind the visor for a deed to Loonie Lake.

"That house isn't large enough for three of us," Shelly said, "and Russell Robins sold mine."

"We'll add wings. Do you want to get married before or after we swing by for your things? I have to make an honest woman out of you."

"Lawyers don't have to be honest, just expedient. And marriage doesn't have

234

anything to do with honesty."

"Then I'll make an expedient woman out of you, but you're not a lawyer any more. You're an EMT with a brand new ambulance and a large enough back-up crew to give you a shot at motherhood. Are we having a boy or a girl?"

"The ultrasound says boy, but what makes you so sure you're the sire? And what makes you think I'd marry you if you were?"

"I counted backward, but I'm doing a DNA anyway, after he comes. Also I entered the date in my notebook the night you heard the alarm buzz on your biological clock."

"Even with that," Shelly said, "the only sure parent is the mother, and I think I'm going to name him Carl, after Dr. Hogue and Buster."

"I don't think *that* will hurt his luck one bit." There was a satisfying justice in my son's becoming the namesake of the end of a line. Growing up in Grady, he'd have something I'd never had until now--a sense of belonging somewhere besides Washington. Nobody belongs in Washington.

I'd like to say that the arguments I'd tediously mapped out to convince Shelly to drop out of law school and marry me won over her heart, but honesty forbids me. She had, as a matter of fact, already withdrawn from Vanderbilt by the time I arrived and was saying her goodbys to the dean, a family friend, at the very moment I charged across campus to rescue her from a disgraceful and unproductive future. She'd realized after six weeks of fellowship with the legally inspired that the ACLU would end up defending the Klan by the time she hung her shingle. During the tenure of her career there promised to be more lawyers than law in the U.S.A., where attorneys would be forced into a form of cannibalistic symbiosis at the top of the food chain, suing each other or advertising on TV for potential malpractice clients--making more laws to accommodate the excess of legal minds to interpret them. The greatest injustice, Shelly decided after the first month of law school, is premature death. Whether I had come for her or not, she'd have continued somewhere, Flint most likely, as an EMT and raised a child named Buster.

I'd never been happier or felt a more absorbing sense of purpose. The new smell of upholstery, the response of 210 horsepower, the knowledge that I was transporting my future wife and son to my future home--home. The urn with Shelly's father's ashes was stowed safely behind the double locked doors of the drug box.

There's a sense of power, I'm sure, that derives from being behind the wheel of some engine of destruction, a tank, say, or a Huey gunship, but that power is nothing like the feeling that comes from cruising at night in a 460 cc gasoline V-8 ambulance with a 4-barrel carburetor--that portable capsule of solace, salvation, order, and deliverance from pain for the desperate and dying. How mindless I had been to underestimate the importance of Shelly's profession. "Pull over," she said, "I'll drive."

Chapter Fifty-Two

There were about eighty people attending the staff meeting in the conference room of Putnam Memorial. Besides the medical staff, select members of the Flint community were invited. I was terrified by the idea of speaking before this group, of requesting hospital privileges for my "boondocks practitioners," as we had come to be called even before my recruits could arrive. Maloy was a far better speaker than I'd ever be, but Shelly said I'd be viewed as less of an outsider in the "good old boy" network. For better or worse, I was an established part of the medical community. It was my place to plead our case. Nancy and Maloy agreed.

Country Trulane, the chief of staff, called the meeting to order: "We have two main orders of business that everybody already knows about. One is a proposal from Dr. Stone from Grady to be accepted on staff along with his partner Dr. Maloy. Drs. Stone and Maloy want to start community health centers in south Flint and in Grady. They'll need a place to hospitalize their patients." Trulane took a long look around the room. "The second is to consider a fundamental restructuring of Putnam Memorial Hospital from a private not-for-profit institution to a private for-profit corporation that will be owned by individual investors, the principal being Karl Wright, who's here to discuss the proposal with you. As is our tradition, we'll let our guests make their presentations first. Dr. Stone?"

Shelly squeezed my hand. I walked to the front of the meeting hall and replaced Country Trulane at the podium. "I appreciate the opportunity to speak to the staff of Putnam Memorial Hospital," I began. "I appreciate the support of the specialists, who have readily accepted the patients I've referred to them. Many of you are not aware of the fact that Trafford Memorial Hospital has been sold to Karl Wright, and it will soon be converted to an outpatient surgery center to specialize in predominantly cataract surgery. I'd hoped to maintain some acute care hospital beds at Trafford, but Mr. Wright informs me that I have one month to arrange for hospitalization of my patients elsewhere. He informs me that my practice doesn't generate enough profit to warrant its continuation." I noticed a few elevated eyebrows and cocked ears, but I couldn't interpret their meaning. "I arrived by accident in Grady," I continued, "never expecting to be a general practitioner in a rural setting such as Grady. I'd planned to practice in a large academic center and to specialize. I could not anticipate the satisfaction that I would receive in providing health care services to the many needy and disadvantaged of Grady County. These are fine, hard-working people who deserve the best medical care that I can provide for them.

"Unfortunately, I cannot follow in the footsteps of my predecessor, Dr.

Hogue; because of his broad training as a family physician he was able to provide pediatric, obstetrical, and general surgery services in addition to the adult medical services that I am now providing. This broader array of services provided a higher hospital census and financial stability. I've tried my best as a general internist to fulfill the needs of the community and to stabilize the hospital. Unfortunately, I have failed in both regards. As you know, an internist thinks a lot and does very little that the insurance companies are willing to pay for. The more skillful he becomes, the more he thinks and the less he does."

This brought some polite laughter. "Dr. Maloy and I have put our heads together with such ironic and lucrative effect that we have all but put ourselves out of business." Nearly everyone smiled. A few doctors laughed sympathetically.

"After extensive consideration," I continued, "I believe the health needs of Grady can only be met through two solutions. The first is through the development of a community health center network that would be housed in Grady and South Flint. These health centers would actually be owned by community boards of directors and receive funding from the U. S. Public Health Service. These additional funds would allow us to see all the indigent people in these two areas and allow us to provide the comprehensive array of services that their poverty and geographic isolation requires. By receiving these funds, these centers will be eligible for placement of National Service Corps personnel. I have already recruited two internists, two pediatricians, and two PAs who'll be coming to join the practice in July, providing you will extend hospital privileges to myself and these future partners. The people of Grady County are depending on your support."

There were the objections Puck Middlebrooks had prepared me for, including the "government doctor" argument and the fiscal impact of dumping more indigent patients into a system that was already delivering $8 million in uncompensated services. Gordon Powell, who sat in the audience between my empty seat and Maloy, had advised me that I had a fair chance of getting the privileges under the present charter, but if the hospital sold out to Wright, I was, of course, dead in the water.

For what it was worth, I assured the medical staff that the doctors I was bringing in had respectable credentials, that they were not going to be eight-to-fivers, and I invited the staff to examine them individually rather than ask for blanket consent. I also announced that I had measured the distance from the shores of Lake Loonie to the halls of Putnam Memorial on the odometer of my now deceased and disintegrated Falcon and had found that I was 23.4 miles away, well within the twenty-five mile limit.

I left the podium and returned to my seat. I couldn't determine how my

238

request had been received. A few of the staff smiled politely. Others nodded affirmatively, but of course it was impossible to know whether they were courteously welcoming me to their meeting or accepting me into their community.

"You were adequate," Shelly assured me when I sat down.

"Adequate?"

Gordon Powell smiled.

"The next decision," Trulane said, regaining the podium, "will be a landmark in the history of Putnam Memorial Hospital. We have to decide whether we continue our current charter, seeing all patients who come to us regardless of their ability to pay, or whether the hospital should be sold to a private corporation and, in essence, become a private, for-profit organization that could include shareholders, possibly some of the physicians in this room. I've discussed this decision with the staff officers, who, as you know, now sit on the Board of Trustees of this hospital. The staff officers include myself as Chief of Staff; Dr. Tom Bovard, who is vice chief; and Dr. Gordon Powell, who is secretary of staff. As you recall, when Mr. Wilson Warwick took over as administrator, he restructured the hospital so that three members of the medical staff, namely its executive committee, would occupy three seats on the seven-member hospital authority. Mr. Karl Wright has been able to initiate a proxy vote in opposition of the hospital administration."

Trulane paused, his eyes slowly scanning the staff. "I should mention," he said, "that this purchase of the hospital would be essentially a hostile takeover since the current administration does not agree with the sale. Within the charter of the hospital authority, however, there is a stipulation that any member of the trustees may produce motions at the trustee meetings and that these motions do not require approval of the chief executive office of the hospital."

Ned Babione, who owned an office supply business and whom Powell described as Wright's mole, had introduced the proposal. "It boils down to this," Powell whispered. "The three staff officers will vote as a block with whatever the majority of the staff votes. Babione plus the staff's three will restructure Putnam into a profit-driven corporation and you have, as they say, shot craps in New Orleans."

"What's *that* mean?" I whispered back.

"It means," he said, "you won't get an uninsured patient within three city blocks of these hallowed halls unless you co-sign his note."

"I want input from all physicians who have something to say," Trulane continued. "We'll stay here all night if necessary, but the hospital board meets at 8:00 a.m. and we'll need your decision by then, so please limit your statements to five minutes. Dr. Gordon, Dr. Bovard, and I will reserve our comments for the end, but now I'm going to ask Mr. Wright to address you. I'm also going to allow him to answer questions concerning his presentation. We will then move to a closed ballot."

Seated between Lee Bob and Beulah Parker was none other than that accomplished health care entrepreneur and sire to a generation of vipers, Karl Wright. He rose and walked to the podium to replace his nephew, kin but not kind. I was a little surprised by how healthful he looked, prosperous, rosy complected, pleasingly obese and well-tailored in his pinstriped Armani with black Gucci loafers and a diamond on his pinkie. I guess I expected him to look ostensibly corrupt and revolting now that I knew his designs. He didn't. He looked benign, successful, and dangerous.

"I appreciate the opportunity to make this historic proposal to the staff at Putnum Memorial. As you are well aware, the challenges facing hospitals these days are monumental. There are continuing cutbacks in reimbursement from private insurance and also federal reimbursement through Medicare and Medicaid. Additionally, there is a progressively larger number of uninsured individuals who will stress the capability of any hospital's survival." Here, Wright drank a long swallow of water, crooking his little finger, flashing cold light.

"The past five years at Putnum reflect this negative trend. Your hospital has declined from maintaining a positive balance of from $1 to $2 million a year to this year, when you have a projected negative cash balance of $1 million. Your open-door policy, while honorable in its intention, is unfortunately unsound in today's business climate." Wright paused, shaking his head sadly as he presumably envisioned Putnum sinking slowly into the fiscal mire. Then he brightened.

"I offer you the opportunity to be purchased by my corporation, which has a very solid management history. We have turned a profit in each of the hospitals that I've acquired. North of here, I currently manage three smaller rural hospitals. Even in this rather unfavorable rural setting, we have been able to amass a profit in excess of $3 million over the past two years. I own other medical facilities and service agencies, including a home health agency and a nursing home that is run by my daughter Beulah and her husband Dr. Parker. I also own and manage Southern Vision, a regional ophthalmology program that features your own chief of staff, Dr. A. Hamilton Trulane. This program has developed into the largest and most profitable outpatient surgery operation in the Southeast."

Wright paused for the vision of his success to be absorbed by the staff. Then he turned to thoughts of the future. "If I can acquire Putnum," he continued. "I will be able to develop a regional network of health services here. This would include outpatient surgery centers, a nursing home, and visiting nursing services.

I also plan to incorporate an array of small rural hospitals that will feed into Putnam. I recently acquired Trafford Memorial Hospital in Grady. Dr. Stone, like most talented and kind-hearted physicians, is a much better doctor than a businessman. The hospital was on the verge of financial collapse, but I was able to save it. Unfortunately, given the nature of physicians practicing in that community, the hospital will have to be changed in the scope of its service and converted to a surgery center, which will be the regional ophthalmology center for the southern tier of our state and which will impact Alabama and Florida.

"If I can acquire Putnam," he repeated, "my accountants project profits that will exceed $10 million next year, and we anticipate greater than a 10% return for your invested dollar. I say *your* because local physicians will be able to invest in my network. In essence, I offer you the opportunity to invest in yourselves, to secure your hospital environment, and to establish a regional health system that is based upon the great American way of doing business . . . ."

"Is it time to wave our flags yet?" whispered Shelly.

"Shsssh," I said.

Carl Gordon smiled supportively. "He's getting ready to say something you may not like," he whispered.

". . . providing excellent services to those who can pay for it, with the forces of the marketplace dictating success or failure. I understand the medical marketplace and know that I can develop a partnership that would maximize returns for myself and for you. I wholeheartedly urge you to join in my efforts."

Wright looked mournfully over the heads of his audience, as though preparing to mouth a truth that pained him deeply and personally. "I sincerely wish we could make our services available to everyone, but this is, as you are painfully aware, a fiscal impossibility. An open door policy will pronounce, as it did with Trafford, doom to the survival of the institution and an unnecessary financial burden upon the taxpayers. I offer you an opportunity to join the future of medicine in this country, and ask you to be bold pioneers, to take the first giant strides necessary to save medicine. Thank you." Karl Wright rejoined Lee Bob and Beulah, who smiled like a barracuda.

"Let's take a ten minute break and return for a question and answer session," said Country Trulane.

We stood up to stretch. "How's little Carl 'Buster' Stone doing?" I asked Shelly, glancing at her hard round belly.

"It's Carl 'Buster' Farmer, and he's rambunctious." She placed her hands into the small of her back and leaned backwards.

"Daddy's little boy," I said, placing my palm on Shelly's abdomen to feel my progeny kick.

"Wright's applying cutthroat free market principles to a system that is ripe for takeover and restructuring," Gordon Powell said. " The hospital will discontinue services that aren't profitable and refuse to serve people who can't pay."

"He won't get away with it will he?" Shelly asked.

"He's got a really good chance," answered Dr. Powell. "He's been buying off key doctors with stock options and sweetheart deals."

"Sweetheart deals?" I asked.

"Sure, he provides you staff and facilities at the center, forgives your rent for a year."

"Is that legal?" The politics of medicine was a whole new area for me.

"It's legal, if not quite ethical," said Dr. Powell.

"What will the public say--they won't stand for this will they?"

"The media will cover the board meeting and report the outrage in three-inch headlines, but by the time it gets public it's a done deal. Corporate raiders like Carl Wright have the financial and legal means to take over a community hospital even before the board meets."

"Doing business the Great American Way," said Jim Maloy.

After the break Dr. Phil Mendenbaum, oncologist, stood up. His perpetual exposure to terminal cancer patients had instilled him with a *carpe diem* attitude that threatened to dissipate him before middle age. A compulsive outdoorsman, he tried to cram four or five lives into one by working and playing harder than anyone else, but he was also among the most willing to provide care for the poor and uninsured. I wasn't surprised that he asked Wright the first question: "What happens to the patients without money that are already in therapy? I'm going to find it difficult morally to discontinue services to dying cancer patients just because they can't pay."

"Good question, Dr. Mendenbaum," Wright said.

"Unfortunately, cancer chemotherapy has had a very negative impact on the cash flow of this hospital. These patients would have to be transferred. I would arrange for outpatient chemotherapy, but the burden for hospitalization would have to be borne by the oncology center at the state hospital in Augusta."

Jeff Roberts stood up. A paradox of medicine and mankind, he wore a black leather Harley Davidson jacket and a pair of scuffed-up Dingo boots. If Hack was an intellectual redneck, Roberts was a philanthropic thug. Although he was the most generous contributor of charity services to my patients, he looked more the type to wield a switchblade than a scalpel. He incarnated the idea that some doctors, like some saints, are chosen by some power or force beyond the human domain. "What happens if a gentlemanly father-of-five presents to the emergency room with an acute myocardial infarction or a ruptured aorta and needs immediate surgery?" It was clear how Roberts felt. It was *always* clear how Roberts felt. He was solidly in favor of the underdog.

"Of course we would have to stabilize some acute traumas before transportation," Wright answered, "but Augusta is only three hours away." Roberts absorbed Wright's answer with stony and contemptuous silence.

Dr. Lawson Odoms, a black OBGYN, spoke next. "As a practicing obstetrician sympathetic to the needs of the minority community, I would find it unconscionable to transport indigent women three hours for delivery. Are you telling me that I will have no decision on who I can and cannot admit to the hospital? I think this would have a disastrous impact on our already unacceptable infant mortality rate." Dr. Odoms, Dr. Roberts, and Dr. Mendenbaum were in favor of keeping the open doors open.

"Although I agree with you," Wright droned, "unless Medicaid is willing to expand its coverage, we simply cannot be available to deliver all women who present. Women who have no insurance will have to be more careful about when and if they become pregnant . . . ."

"Would you listen to that pluperfect son-of-a-bitch?" Shelly said loud enough for everybody within a three-row vicinity to hear. I cringed.

". . . as you are well aware," he continued, "we have a very unacceptable rate of teenage pregnancy and unwed mothers. I have contacted Augusta and St. Mary's Home for Unwed Mothers in Augusta, and they have agreed to house women in the last two months of their pregnancies. They will be delivered at Augusta, and the children can be adopted there or the mothers can bring them home with them."

Odoms was still shaking his head when a Dr. Hofstetter asked how much Putnam would save by transferring its indigent care to Augusta, where the taxpayers have already agreed to pay for it. "Would this balance our budget?"

"Thank you, Dr. Hofstetter. Currently, this hospital is delivering around $8 million in uncompensated services," Wright said. "By transporting our indigent patients, we will be able to net a profit of over $5 million next year. Also, with our marketing skills, we should be able to attract paying customers throughout the region and improve the cash flow of your own practices in the hospital."

Dr. Odoms wanted to have Wilson Warwick, the hospital administrator, address the meeting, but since the proposal amounted to a hostile takeover that would remove Warwick from the management structure, the board moved for a resolution for proxy requesting that Warwick not address this body since such an address would constitute a conflict of interest. We took another short break before the grand old men, Powell, Bovard, and Trulane made statements. Shelly went to the ladies' room. She said Little Carl was working out on her bladder like a speedbag.

"The longer this goes on," Gordon Powell told me, "the more visceral it will become. People get tired, they use their guts instead of their brains."

"It's well orchestrated," observed Maloy. "They've been working this out for a long time."

"Oh yes. If they hadn't thought they had it sewn up, they wouldn't have risked the motion," Powell said.

"How will the younger docs vote?" Nancy asked.

"They'll go with the flow," said Powell. "They're waiting to see how the *old* boys lean. They realize they haven't been around long enough to understand how hospital politics affects them financially."

"I thought doctors knew everything the moment they graduated med school," said Nancy ironically, "from flying airplanes to investing in the stock market. The last course in the medical curriculum is called Comprehensive Life Skills, where they learn how to exit a sand trap and draw to an inside straight."

Powell smiled, "In politics and business talented young doctors are the most innocent creatures God has invented since the fall of Eden."

Nancy giggled at Shelly, who'd returned from the bathroom and overheard Powell. She was cutting her eyes in my direction and was pointing to me with both thumbs and her tongue.

"They have strong liberal arts and science backgrounds as undergraduates," Powell continued, "simply because med schools don't accept business and political science majors. During med school, internship, and residency, they're taught that the business end of their practice is a dangerous and unholy mixture and are advised to hire business managers to handle the dirty work of fiscal health. Wright's goods are tempting because he's telling them, go ahead, read your journals and keep up in your fields, just keep being good doctors and let me make sure you have a nice hospital. I'll see to it that you pay off your $80,000 med school debt and keep up your $30,000 malpractice premiums."

"They don't know owl shit from Oil of Olay," Shelly reiterated.

"What will you say when it's your turn to speak," Nancy asked Powell.

The black surgeon, an old military man and a veteran politician, smiled sadly. "Oh, I'll say that health care is a fundamental human right, not a privilege for the wealthy. I'll speak of Hippocrates, and basic obligations a doctor has to alleviate human suffering. I'll talk of the horror of premature babies born in hospital parking lots, of white haired grandmothers with terminal cancer that has spread to the liver, of the agony of the ischemic gut, of leaking aneurysms, of spiculated kidney stones, fractured femurs, ruptures, tubal pregnancy, perforated ulcers, ruptured discs, and testicular torsion. I'll plead for human decency, and I'll saw the air with my hands. I will win the hearts of this audience." He shook his head, resigned. "But I will not win their vote."

"You sound cynical, Gordon Powell." This from Nancy.

"Only realistic, my dear. The other doctors expect me and Dr. Odoms to strongly favor the open door since we're black and the majority of indigent patients who'll be turned away will be black too. My theatrics will prick their consciences, but Wright knows I can't swing the vote. He's waited for the right moment to make his move, and he's got Dr. Bovard, who's been on the staff of this hospital for 40 years. Bovard's a very strong politician locally and with the AMA. He'll deliver an eloquent prophesy of doom argument against the open door policy. He'll assert that a hospital that isn't sensitive to the economic climate will fail, as Trafford did, and that open-door policies are no longer financially viable in the existing economic climate. He'll insist that the medical students at Augusta need these indigents to practice and train on. and he'll charge us with the task of responsible stewardship of the Flint community's only hospital."

"What about Dr. Trulane?" Maloy asked. "Is he a good guy or a bad guy."

"We're all good guys," Dr. Gordon said, "even Karl Wright, who is a good businessman applying sound economic principles to make Putnam fiscally sound. Doctors deserve super-adequate compensation for their commitment and training and need it to survive in a parasitic ecosystem, where a malpractice attorney lurks around every bush, but Trulane is Wright's trump card, his ace in the hole."

"Will Trulane speak out in favor of the takeover?"

"He won't have to. Trulane's one of the most highly respected ophthalmologists in the Southeast, he's Chief of staff, and he's Karl Wright's nephew, whom Wright raised and educated. The staff will approve the takeover in deference to Trulane's blood. You're still in the South, young doctor. Dr. Trulane's silence will be his consent."

Chapter Fifty-Three

The meeting continued as if Gordon Powell had written the script. He delivered a moving auditory that inspired applause, even a standing ovation from nearly half of those in attendance. Then came Dr. Bovard's stern charge that the doctors' responsibility was to keep the hospital alive by whatever practical means available. "We are the stewards of health for Southwest Georgia," he concluded. "We can not save those who have fallen overboard by sinking the ship." He too got a standing ovation, a considerably louder one than Gordon Powell's.

"Well, that about does it," said Powell. "A good politician doesn't call for the motion until he knows it will carry."

"It's time to call in the dogs and piss on the fire," said Maloy, miming the voice of Hack Singletree. The staff was restless; it was getting late. Tired voters lean toward maintaining the status quo.

But Country Trulane surprised us. He returned to the podium, asking that the staff indulge him to say a few brief words of a personal nature before the guests were excused and cleared for the balloting.

"I owe much to Karl Wright," he began, "my uncle."

"Talk about overkill," said Jim Maloy, crossing his long legs.

"Wait a minute," said Powell, touching Jim's arm.

"He paid for my medical training, and he helped me to establish my ophthalmology program here in Southwest Georgia," Trulane continued. "Through his brilliant financial guidance, I was able to realize a net income in excess of $750,000 last year, which put me, according to *Medical Economics*, in the top 1% of the nation's physicians as far as income is concerned. This represents a very successful marketing of my skills, the kind of marketing that Uncle Karl is capable of, and I was, until very recently, smugly satisfied that I was doing my part for the service of humankind and making a damn good living at the same time. I smiled at myself as I shaved, and I whistled on the way to work, secure in knowing I was a good doctor who gave better health to virtually everybody I saw."

Here Trulane paused so long it seemed he'd forgotten the content of his message. "Spending one day in Dr. Stone's office made me realize the impact the closed doors of my medical practice were having on community health. I was curing everybody I saw because I was seeing the curable. Victims of poverty and long-term medical neglect got screened out by my secretaries, receptionists, and business managers. Uncle Karl had skillfully marketed my talents, and he had thrown in my soul as a bonus." He smiled sadly, looking around the room. "Remember doctors, there is an M.D. after your name, not an M.B.A. Your sworn duty is to serve. Profit must never replace service. Please join me in rejecting the proxy."

"Well I'll be damned," smiled Gordon Powell, absolutely out of character. "I'll be double-dog damned."

Chapter Fifty-Four

I've got something to show you," Country Trulane told me, rushing into my office with a calfskin briefcase hugged to his chest, not trusting the grip. He was bubbling over, and his mood was all the richer because I'd never seen him thrilled about anything.

I'd just returned from a grand jury subpoena. Morton Willetts got Wilkin acquitted on Rooster's DUI charge on the basis of my reluctant testimony that Wilkin Wright was diabetic and prone to hypoglycemia, a condition that causes staggering and confusion. My insistence that Wilkin was *drunk* when he killed Ethel Hargrove--that his diabetes was incidental--almost got me cited for contempt. It was beginning to look like Wilkin couldn't find a better friend than he had in me.

It was the second time I'd gone to the courthouse that week. I'd driven Hack to the courthouse to answer Karl Wright's charges that he'd planted a four-foot cottonmouth moccasin *Akistron, Pisciverous, pisciverous* as thick as a link of bologna into the window of Wilkin Wright's new Mazda. The snake's beaded head appeared between Wilkin's feet as the Mazda sped down 85, and Wilkin abandoned the vehicle about the same time it banjoed through Billy Mack Halliburton's barbed wire fence.

"When Rooster gets done dusting that snake for fingerprints," Hack grinned balefully, "y'all will doubtless conclude my innocence or guilt, but till then if I was you, I'd check my mail with a flashlight." Of course the evidence had either crawled off or was still somewhere in the Mazda, which had been towed to Melvin's garage because nobody would drive it. It sat next to Miss Ethel's Buick for the time being, since nobody was anxious to get his face close enough to look under the seat either. It was a matter of much dispute as to whether the musky smell in the car was residual or active.

"That dopehead hallucinated that snake in the first place," Hack told the judge. Then his smile melted as he arcwelded his gaze on Wilkin, who shuffled his feet and sawed his eyes. Hack's lost weight made him look even meaner, the way a bulldog's sagging jowls add to its air of tenacity. Going without whiskey hadn't improved his disposition, either. "You ever tried to get juiced on embalming fluid, boy?" he asked Wilkin. "No matter what you up on, I guaran-goddamn-tee you that stuff can bring you down."

"That constitutes a threat, Judge," Karl Wright protested.

"That constitutes a question," Rooster answered.

"That constitutes a damned *suggestion*," Hack hissed, flashing his lower incisors, "that you keep your boy's maloccluded ass on the far side of the Grady County line while he can still push a reading on a rectal thermometer."

"Order!" said Judge Savage.

———————

The impetus for Trulane's blithe spirits was, of course, a snake-eye disk, more artfully conceived than any of the other three, but identical in motif except for the bright eye in the palm, which was inlaid with quartz crystal. He was as happy as I've ever seen a grown man. "Did you have anything to do with it, Otis?"

"Nothing whatever."

"It was delivered to my office in a pickup with a Grady County tag registered to Maynard Hullet," he said. "My receptionist had gone in early to help me with the transition from Southern Vision. She thought the driver was trying to burglarize the place and jotted down his tag number. The police traced it for us. Do you know Hullet?"

"Sure, he's a patient of mine."

"He's not an Indian, is he?"

"No, but he's got some red skin around his neck," I said. "Frog Hullet's a gofer for some people around Grady who want to keep their identity anonymous. You won't find out anything from him. The disk didn't come from Frog."

I walked Country Trulane out to his Jaguar, which looked quite elegant parked on the Savannah brick pavement of my parking lot, its deeply lacquered finish reflecting the leaves of my live oak. Patients in the brick gazebo and in the walled-in garden enjoyed the spring sunshine until Early May called them in to be prepped by my new office nurse Margaret Holt.

"There's never been a snake-eye disk with quartz inlay before," Trulane said. "At least I've never heard of one."

"Well, you deserve to have one then."

"What for?"

"For your part in getting my staff hospital privileges at Putnam and for making the scales fall from an old man's eyes."

Trulane's mouth dropped open. His eyes widened. "Kinnard!" he exclaimed, his hand slapping his forehead. "The old Indian made the disks. It never occurred to me the snake/eye artist might still be alive."

"He's alive," I said. "And if I were you, I wouldn't wander unannounced down in the Toa to express my gratitude. He's a crack shot now that he's not blind. He might fire a bullet through you before you get close enough to recognize."

"Well, I'll be damned," said Trulane. "I'll just be damned."

Karl Wright had predictably severed all ties with his nephew, and Trulane had gone in with another ophthalmologist for the time being. The looks Karl and Beulah gave Country as they left the staff meeting could have freeze dried a watermelon, but I decided that the best known ophthalmologist in southwest Georgia wasn't in any immediate danger of starving. Indigent and uninsured patients, historically receiving poor or no optical health care, now had access to the best. Our most fervent disciple of a comprehensive quality health care system for the underserved, Trulane had been spreading the word that 20% reduction in income could buy doctors back the peace of mind they'd lost when they started turning their backs on patients who weren't lucrative. "So I die with $2.5 million in the bank instead of $3 million," he told potential converts to the system.

We were startled by three long blasts from a horn, and Hack's battered green pickup, trailing smoke, rattled up with Mary Lou peeking through the steering wheel. Hack rode shotgun, waving a big hand and grinning with teeth made even more equine with his loss of weight.

Mary Lou had followed Hack home from Putnam and moved in to help him bathe and don his support hose. She made large pots of angelica tea to keep him dry. She also drove him to his speed reading classes and AA meetings, where Maloy worried that Hack would swap his alcohol addiction for a caffeine and donut dependency. He had recovered quickly from his heart attack and bypass surgery.

Nancy had come up with the idea that Hack's print addiction would be less of a nuisance if his reading speed could be accelerated beyond 250 words per minute, the speed that people read aloud. This, she reasoned, would eliminate his infuriating habit of reading road signs. His mind, she reasoned, would process the next message before his mouth could frame the words.

Shelly, who treated Hack more like a benign cancer than the plague now that he was the property of Mary Lou, said the course would make him worse. He'd just read aloud much faster to keep up.

Initially Hack objected to going to AA. He said that he didn't like the idea of making new friends whose sole personal qualification was a history of substance abuse. "You dumb son-of-a-bitch," Shelly countered, "that's the way you've made friends all your sorry-assed life." We all wondered what would happen if Wilkin Wright ever joined Hack's group, which dealt with narcotic abuse as well as alcohol.

Hack and Mary Lou brought glad tidings. "Look in the back," they said. On a blanket of hay in the bed of his truck Syndrome lay on her side. Nine hairless pink piglets fought for teats as the mother grunted proudly, her porcine mouth turned up at the corners. Hack shook Country Trulane's hand after Trulane thrust it into the open window of the truck. I scratched Syndrome behind the ear. "How?" I asked.

"How'd you think?" squeaked Mary Lou. "The angels brung them or the stork?" She jumped out of the cab.

"But she was sequestered in an electric fence," I exclaimed.

"What we got here," said Hack, "is a Catholic who don't believe in virgin birth."

I'd never seen new born piglets before.

"Ain't they cute?" said Mary Lou, who was standing on tiptoes to see over the tailgate.

"Did you have her bred or what?"

"Naw, a feral hog broke through. Big black razorback. I heard them getting it on. They sounded like wore out brakes on a freight train. Then the boar busted back out, leaving Miss Syndrome in a family way."

Shelly finally agreed to marry me, and we set the date for Sunday, June 17, two weeks before the recruited doctors for our clinics were slated to arrive. Puck Middlebrooks assured us that although we'd be cutting it closer than most shotgun weddings, we'd be back from our honeymoon with at least four weeks to spare before Carl arrived. Middlebrooks should have known by now that Shelly was famous for jumping the gun.

Father Flannery, in an unprecedented ecumenical event, came in from Flint to perform the service in the sanctuary of the Grady Methodist Church. A gaunt Hack Singletree was best man. Jim Maloy, Country Trulane, and J. Puckett Middlebrooks ushered. Mary Lou, who looked like a flower girl, joined Nancy, Early May, and Cyrilla Hargrove as bridesmaids. Margaret Holt, matron of honor, followed her protuberant bottom lip down the aisle like a Moorish warrior in purple taffeta. Dr. Paul Dudley gave the bride away, and Dr. Gordon Powell gave his blessings. We all felt that the celebration joined more than me and Shelly. And Miss Ida actually cried, a phenomenon even her husband Bill said he'd never witnessed.

Shelly and I hurried through a blizzard of rice to Country Trulane's Jaguar. I helped her into the low bucket seat and strapped her in, precious cargo. We planned to drive to Saint Simons, a barrier island on the Georgia coast, where Jeff Roberts, Gordon Powell, and Puck Middlebrooks had chipped in for reservations at the honeymoon suite of the Cloister Hotel.

I brushed rice out of Shelly's hair, which she'd let grow out nearly to her shoulders to celebrate matrimony and motherhood, I thought, although she insisted she let it grow every winter. I noticed that some of the rice appeared finely ground into minute particles, some of which had gotten in her ear. "Those bastards were throwing grits!" I exclaimed.

I cranked the Jaguar--or tried to. The engine turned over with enthusiastic battery but impotent spark. The car curse was still upon me. "Shit," I said, my first expression of frustration within the context of conjugal bliss.

Melvin sidled over. "You hell on internal combustion machinery, ain't you Doc?"

The wedding guests howled, slinging more rice and grits. Mary Lou did a series of cartwheels and a back flip. Her panties were white, matching her organdy dress. She had, of course, caught the bridal bouquet. Elroy Singletree watched her, grinning mindlessly and clapping his hands.

"Better pull the hood," Melvin said. He pushed up the sleeves of his sport coat and reattached the plug wires Puck Middlebrooks had disconnected. Melvin slammed the hood and ran to the wrecker to chase us out of town.

The Jag cleared its throat and growled, barking rubber as I U-turned and headed east. The motorcade, led by Rooster Bootman's patrol car, the new ambulance, and Melvin's wrecker disturbed the peace with multitone sirens and flashing lights all the way to the county line, where they stopped and turned back toward Grady. The late afternoon sun through the rear window irradiated Shelly's hair and cast her face in partial shadow as we headed east across the coastal plains to the sea. Her eyes were bright with joy and maternity. One ear glowed red, incandescent with magnified sunlight. "Well Stone," she said, resting her hand on the top of my thigh, "do you think you can get there from here?"

"Stick with me," I urged. "I can take us there, and I can bring us back. I've newly acquired an inexplicable and faultless sense of direction."

"Well, see if you can turn this Jaguar around and find your way back to the clinic," she laughed. "My water just broke."

(end)